"Great writing about grief is all too rare. In this book you will journey with people who have faced incredible losses—the kinds most of us don't even want to think about: people who have lost loved ones to cancer, heart attacks, car accidents, plane crashes, suicide, and even murder. Yet despite unbelievable grief and distress, each found a God who cared and was present. This is an essential book for all who have suffered a loss—I guess that means everyone."

JAMES A. AVERY, M.D.
Medical director, Visiting Nurse Service of New York Hospice Care; assistant clinical professor, Mount Sinai School of Medicine

"Lynn Eib weaves together a magnificent patchwork of grievers' stories with the golden thread of the powerful testimony of God's words. If you're so brokenhearted you don't know if you'll survive—if your soul is so parched it feels as if it's cracking and turning to dust—if you've cried to the point that your tear glands feel as if they've dried up, don't miss the soothing and healing balm in this wonderful book. When God and grief meet, true healing can begin."

WALT LARIMORE, M.D.
Award-winning medical journalist; coauthor of *His Brain, Her Brain*

"When you're grieving, it helps to spend time with other people who've been there—people who understand the very real fears, disappointments, and sorrow that you are going through. In *When God & Grief Meet*, Lynn Eib introduces us to a series of people who not only share their stories of grief but who offer us wise insights and practical ideas for getting through it."

NANCY GUTHRIE
Author of *Holding On to Hope* and coauthor of *When Your Family's Lost a Loved One*

"*When God & Grief Meet* is a poignant collection of heartwarming real-life stories of those who have found the significance of spirituality in searching for guidance through their grief journeys. This book is a valuable resource to address the most challenging questions one experiences following the loss of a loved one. Lynn has, once again, through the stories of others found comforting words to create peace at this most difficult time in life. I wholly endorse this very valuable grieving tool."

JUDY LENTZ, R.N., M.S.N.
Chief executive officer, Hospice and Palliative Nurses Association

"Grief is hard and lonely work, but in these compelling stories and honest reflections from Lynn Eib, you will find a community of people who understand your sorrow and a God who restores your hope."

HAROLD G. KOENIG, M.D.
Professor of psychiatry and behavioral sciences; associate professor of medicine; codirector, Center for Spirituality, Theology and Health, Duke University Medical Center

"The price of human caring is grief and loss. Whatever one's present state of loss, Lynn provides the reader with an understanding of the grief process and how the application of an active faith can help one live through troubled times. The gift of this book to someone in need will make all the difference."

ROY SMITH, M.DIV., PH.D.
Licensed psychologist; president, Pennsylvania Counseling Services

"Once again Lynn Eib takes readers on a peace-seeking journey with God as the guide. Lynn masterfully takes on the difficult but universally prevalent subject of grief. Her words will resonate with you and comfort you long after you've finished the book."

JULIE K. SILVER, M.D.
Assistant professor, Harvard Medical School; author of *What Helped Get Me Through*

When God & Grief Meet

TRUE STORIES OF COMFORT & COURAGE

LYNN EIB

Author of *When God & Cancer Meet*

TYNDALE
MOMENTUM

An Imprint of
Tyndale House Publishers, Inc.

Visit Tyndale online at www.tyndale.com.

Visit Tyndale Momentum online at www.tyndalemomentum.com.

TYNDALE is a registered trademark of Tyndale House Publishers, Inc. *Tyndale Momentum* and the Tyndale Momentum logo are trademarks of Tyndale House Publishers, Inc. Tyndale Momentum is an imprint of Tyndale House Publishers, Inc.

Library of Congress Cataloging-in-Publication Data

Eib, Lynn.
    When God & grief meet : true stories of comfort and courage / Lynn Eib.
        p. cm.
    ISBN 978-1-4143-2174-5 (sc)
    1. Consolation. 2. Bereavement—Religious aspects—Christianity. 3. Grief—Religious aspects—Christianity. I. Title.
    BV4905.3.E35 2009
    248.8′66—dc22   2008031034

Printed in the United States of America

20   19   18   17   16   15   14
10   9   8   7   6   5   4

To my husband—

In the words of Joe Wise:
I'm in love with my God
My God's in love with me.
And the more I love you
the more I know,
I'm in love with my God.
I'm forever grateful
I was part of God's plan
to turn your
mourning into joy.

CONTENTS

ACKNOWLEDGMENTS

Every time I finish writing another book, I am *sure* it will be my last. And then God puts another book inside my head and I have to write again. I can tell you that without His supernatural touch, I would have had nothing of eternal value to say. If anything in this book comforts your heart, please give Him all the credit.

I also would like to say **thank you** to:

My prayer partner and dear friend, **Elizabeth Hirsh**, for praying me through all my writing and expertly editing my manuscript so I look much better to my publisher.

My husband's prayer partner and my dear friend, **Dr. Marc Hirsh**, for giving me a job that allows me to share the Lord with so many suffering and grieving people (and for not retiring yet!).

All the members of my **Grief Prayer Support Group** for allowing me to test some of my book ideas on them and for entrusting me with their grief-storms.

All **the grievers in this book** for unselfishly sharing their stories with the hope they might encourage others.

My Haitian friends in Christ, **Johanne Phanord and Danny Perez**, for assisting me with interviewing Elza Phanord and translating her comments.

My cousin **retired USAF Major James Perkins** for explaining how to fly into the eye of a hurricane (and come out alive).

Therapist **Rebecca Rice** for reviewing some of my psychology comments and making sure I knew what I was talking about even though I'm not a psychologist.

All the wonderful folks at the Knox Group of Tyndale House, especially: associate publisher **Jan Long Harris** for first suggesting I consider writing this book, author relations manager **Sharon Leavitt** for supporting my ministry with her fervent prayers, and editor **Kim Miller** for expertly improving my manuscript.

And most important, my family for loving me and cheering me on: my husband, **Ralph**; my daughter **Bethany** and her husband, **Josh**; my daughter **Danielle Joy**; and my daughter **Lindsey** and her *new,* wonderful husband, **Frank**. (Please note: Now that I have three books, each daughter has had a turn to be mentioned *first*—whew! Hopefully, my sons-in-law are not as competitive and won't demand equal time.)

And, of course, my parents, **Robert and Gaynor Yoxtheimer**, for giving me such a great start in life and for living long enough to see my writing success!

1

Trusting the Magnetic Poles of the Earth

Let's be honest: I never wanted to write a grief book and you never wanted to need one.

Frankly, I like movies with happy endings, fairy tales where everyone lives happily ever after, and answered prayers for miracle healings. But right now you and I are past all those hopes and dreams. Instead we are faced with harsh reality.

I don't know your exact circumstances. Perhaps this enemy called Death snuck up and unexpectedly stole away your loved one. Or perhaps you had been expecting its arrival for some time. Either way it was an unwelcome intruder which brought the ending you never wanted to see.

So I *do* understand that you'd rather not be in the position to *need* this book. But if you picked it up for yourself, I'm honored you have chosen to take my words along with you on your grief journey. If someone gave you this book, I'm praying you'll be just curious enough about what will happen when God meets your grief that you'll keep reading. And if you're not quite ready to read yet, that's okay with me. Just put the book aside (hopefully on the top of your pile!). I believe that sometime in the coming weeks you'll know you're ready. I'll still be here for you then.

It might seem strange for me to say I didn't want to write this book. After all, I am a journalist, and writing normally gives me great joy. I write and speak mostly on the topic of faith and medicine, drawing on my years of experience as a patient advocate offering emotional and spiritual support to cancer patients and their caregivers. As a longtime cancer survivor myself—I was diagnosed with advanced colon cancer at the age of thirty-six in 1990—I love working in my oncologist's office encouraging those facing this dreaded disease. It *can* be a very sad job because more than half our patients die from their cancer. But at least some become survivors, and there's always a glimmer of hope that even those with dire prognoses might defy the odds.

With grief, there's no such glimmer. Nothing I write will change the reality of the loss you are mourning—which is why I was reluctant to write this book. But while my words can't change your past, I believe these true stories from others' grief-storms will give you comfort in your present and courage for your future.

These stories come from people of all walks of life

who have experienced many kinds of difficult losses. Some have lost loved ones to cancer and heart attacks; others have had their worlds ripped apart by a car accident, a plane crash, a suicide, and even a murder. I have no doubt you'll find at least one person facing a grief-storm who has feelings very similar to yours.

The focus of the stories is *not* on how the loved ones died but on how those left behind are finding the strength to continue living without them. My hope is that these stories will help heal your heartache as much as they have mine.

I started feeling especially helpless dealing with grief a few years ago as I watched a march of mourning people come to my office searching for answers, direction, and peace after their loved ones passed away. Many had attended my Cancer Prayer Support Groups with their loved ones and really missed the encouragement those groups offered them. I kept sensing God asking me to start a similar group for grievers, but if you've read my other books, you know I'm not always eager to say yes to the hard things God calls me to do. (If you haven't read my books, let's just say I tend to think I have things all figured out and can convince the Almighty my way is right!)

Starting a grief group sounded *really* depressing to me. Granted, starting a cancer support group sounded *really* depressing to me back in 1991, and it turned out to be an incredible joy, but I was certain this time that a grief group *definitely* would be depressing.

Yet the march of mourners continued to come through my office door, and I found myself spending more and more time each day offering comfort and consolation. I also was having a harder time dealing with my own grief as the deaths of my patient-friends began to add up. Every week another one would die; sometimes a couple of friends would pass in the same day.

God kept tugging on my heart, and I finally asked my boss, Dr. Marc Hirsh, if it would be okay for me to start a grief group at the office. I could tell he really didn't see the necessity of such a gathering, but if I wanted to do it, he wouldn't say no.

So I sent out notes to my grieving friends, inviting them to come to a group meeting at our office. Bringing a bunch of sorrowful souls together in the same room still seemed like a depressing plan—especially because I was powerless to change their painful reality.

But I almost had forgotten that Someone else was going to show up. From the very first grief group, it was obvious to me that God was going to do something special in our midst. Sure, there were plenty of tissues and tear-filled memories, but there also were laughs and comfort-filled words. Instead of being depressed by hearing each other's stories, we all felt just a little bet-ter as we realized we weren't quite so alone. Instead of drowning in our own self-pity, grievers reached out, as if we were throwing life preservers to one another. And instead of feeling far from God, we began to sense His love was very near.

Now, more than five years after that first meeting, the grief group members enjoy each other so much that we also meet monthly for breakfast and dinner and have gotten together for picnics, shows, and concerts. An evening group has been added for those who can't come during the day. And my boss thinks facilitating our ministry to grievers is one of the more important things I do in the office and one of the best ways our patients' families can continue to see God meet their greatest needs.

So my prayer for you as you read these pages is that you'll feel as if you've been to some really good support group meetings. You'll have to add great snacks and jokes if you want them to be more like our group. (Yes, I said jokes. I start every meeting with them because I have found that grievers usually haven't had much to smile about and need a safe place to learn to laugh again.)

You can "go" to a support group meeting once a day, once a week, or once a month depending on how quickly you read this book. You'll know what the right pace is for you. (And if you just can't put the book down, go ahead and have a marathon meeting—but after you finish you'll probably want to come back now and then to give the words a chance to really soak in.)

As we walk this grief journey together, I think you'll discover that many others share your deep feelings. And while I can appreciate the popular psychology that feelings are "neither right nor wrong," I also know that feelings do not necessarily mirror God's undeniable truth.

I witnessed this dilemma of strong feelings at odds with facts a few years ago when my husband and I were out on a boat with my boss, Marc, and his wife, Elizabeth.

The four of us had set out for our annual Labor Day weekend cruise on their thirty-two-foot Bayliner, despite rather foul-looking weather. We were headed up the Chesapeake Bay to a scenic, lively marina called Skipjack Cove on the Sassafras River of Maryland's eastern shore. Elizabeth had checked with her brother who lives right on the Gunpowder River leading into the Chesapeake, and he had assured us the weather reports didn't look that bad, despite a hurricane that was heading northward up the coast. (We later learned he had accidentally listened to the *wrong* forecast.)

So we took off, knowing that Marc and Elizabeth were seasoned boaters—although the whitecaps on the usually calm river should have been our first clue it wasn't a good idea.

We had a short two-hour cruise ahead of us, but it wasn't long before the whitecaps turned into three-foot waves. The wind whipped up, and then the thunder, lightning, and rain came. At first we all laughed and enjoyed the warm rain soaking us as the boat pounded through the waves. But then I stopped laughing, and my stomach started rebelling. Elizabeth handed me a supply of Ziploc bags, which I started filling. The waves were now five feet high and crashing clear over the top of the boat's windshield, drenching us. It was nearly impossible for Marc to see out of the rain-splattered windshield, and my husband and Elizabeth were trying to read the navigational charts and look for the numbered buoys, which would keep us in the correct channel away from large shipping vessels, shallow water, and crab pots. We were too far out to turn back toward home, yet not sure we could make it to our planned destination.

And then it got really bad.

Marc announced that according to the boat's compass we were headed in exactly the wrong direction: south when we should have been heading north.

The rest of us were sure we hadn't turned around— Elizabeth was especially positive we were still pointing in the right direction. She was convinced she would have noticed if the boat had made an about-face. From past experience, I knew she usually was right whenever the two of them had a disagreement about boating.

The three of us looked at Marc, waiting to see what he would do. (Well, I didn't look long because I was busy praying there were enough Ziploc bags.)

After a long pause, Marc posed his now-famous question: "Should I trust my wife . . . or the magnetic poles of the earth?"

It wouldn't have surprised me if he'd gone with Elizabeth's feelings because she was so adamant about them, but his scientific brain won out and Marc made a 180-degree turn with the boat.

Within a few moments, we sighted buoys, confirming

that we, indeed, had been going in the wrong direction despite all of us "feeling" otherwise.

The storm raging around us had distorted reality, and our feelings had fallen fickle.

The same thing can happen in the storms of grief. We can *feel* as if we are completely alone or without purpose or unable to cope. These are the times we need a compass—something that always will steer us in the right direction. Don't worry; I'm not suggesting that I'll be your compass. After half a century of living, I continue to be directionally challenged. (My husband still cringes when he recalls that I once described Spain as being to "the left" of Germany!) Besides, you probably don't need one more helpful person in your life telling you what you *should* (or *shouldn't*) be doing.

What I am suggesting is that the God of the universe has a special affinity for brokenhearted people, and His words are the perfect compass for grievers. A magnetic compass always will point you to the North Pole, and God's Word *always* will point you to His unchanging truths and promises.

> *The Lord is close to the brokenhearted; he rescues those whose spirits are crushed.* Psalm 34:18

> *He heals the brokenhearted and bandages their wounds.* Psalm 147:3

As our "group" facilitator, it's not going to be my job to try and solve your problems. I can't change the reality of your loved one's death—no one can. But I hope to show or perhaps remind you that a deeper spiritual reality transcends our earthly reality. I'll do it by pointing to God's Word as your compass of undeniable truth. If you already think of the Bible as your guide to life, I know you'll appreciate these tender reminders. But if you've not seriously given God's Word central importance in your life, I hope you'll give it a try now. You really have nothing to lose and everything to gain.

> *I weep with sorrow; encourage me by your word.*
> PSALM 119:28

> *When doubts filled my mind, your comfort gave me renewed hope and cheer.* PSALM 94:19

And the truth of that second verse is the reason I decided I would write this book I never wanted to write —because God *can* supernaturally comfort and bring renewed hope and even cheer to those whose minds are filled with doubts and whose hearts are filled with grief.

If you want a book by a psychological expert, you'll have to find an author with a lot more initials after his or her name than I have. If you want in-depth theological answers to the questions of suffering and dying, you'll need to locate some of the resources I've listed in the back of this book. But if you want someone to ride with you in your grief-storm and read the compass, then I'm your person. For some reason that only God knows, I believe He has entrusted me with a message for mourners. And as I share with you God's words to the brokenhearted, I believe you will see that when God and grief meet, His power, peace, and presence are bigger and more real than our uncertainties, sorrow, and loneliness. He is able to be our guiding compass.

> *The LORD will guide you continually, giving you water when you are dry and restoring your strength.*
> ISAIAH 58:11

> *The LORD says, "I will guide you along the best pathway for your life. I will advise you and watch over you."*
> PSALM 32:8

> *Your word is a lamp to guide my feet*
> *and a light for my path. . . .*
> *I have suffered much, O LORD;*
> *restore my life again as you promised.*
> PSALM 119:105, 107

Like Marc as he captained our boat during that stormy trip, it's your choice whether or not to trust the magnetic poles of the earth.

TAKE COMFORT: Grief may distort reality, but there is a deeper spiritual reality that always can be trusted.

FEELING YOUR WORLD FALL APART

It's amazing how quickly your world can fall apart. One minute life seems really good, and the next minute you're wondering how you ever will survive. On a big scale, events like Pearl Harbor, President Kennedy's assassination, and 9/11 remind us that life is precarious. (On a much smaller scale, one minute you're laughing in the summer rain on a boat ride and the next minute you're leaning over a plastic bag!)

Serious illness and death have the ability to shake our worlds unlike anything else.

I never have trouble remembering the year Dot and Conrad Songster's world fell apart because it was the same year mine did too. In March 1990, two of their sons were involved in a serious car accident, and then three months later, I was diagnosed with a serious cancer. Why one of their boys and I both are still alive is a question way too difficult for me to answer. Why their middle son lost his life just when it seemed it was really beginning is far beyond my comprehension.

But what I do know—and my friends Dot and Conrad are living proof of this truth—is that even though you'll never get over your grief, you can get through it.

The trip to Gaithersburg, Maryland, from their home on the southern tier of New York State was supposed to be a great father-son time as Conrad and his youngest son, Tim, nineteen, drove down to visit his middle son, Rick, twenty-two, at Rick's new post-college home. The past year had been a terrific one for all the Songster family. Eldest son Jeff, twenty-four, came home from a four-year stint proudly serving in the U.S. Army. Rick graduated with honors from Clarion University in Pennsylvania and landed a promising job in artificial intelligence with IBM. Tim was a freshman with an appointment to the U.S. Air Force Academy in Colorado Springs. Both Tim and Rick had excelled in national swimming and diving competitions. The hard part of raising three boys was done, and each son was proving that his parents' love and devotion had paid off. Dot and Conrad would, of course, continue to pray daily for their sons, but they breathed a sigh of relief that all three were living productive lives.

Conrad had no special agenda for his weekend with Rick and Tim other than to celebrate Rick's new beginning and enjoy time with his sons. The boys knew from a lifetime of living with their dad that his contribution to their special time would include plenty of dumb jokes,

witty comments, and belly laughs. It was impossible
to spend more than five minutes with him and not be
chuckling—or at least groaning at his quirky sense of
humor. They felt blessed to call him Dad, and Conrad
certainly felt equally blessed to call them his own.

All seemed right with the world.

The world-shattering call came to Conrad from a
Bethesda, Maryland, hospital at about 4 a.m. He was
sleeping at Rick's apartment, unaware the boys hadn't
returned from sightseeing in the area.

"There's been an accident. Can you come to the hospital right away?" the voice queried.

Conrad jerked from his sleep and jumped into his car.
As he pulled out of the apartment parking lot, he realized he didn't even know where the hospital was, but for
some reason a police car appeared suddenly, and Conrad
was able to ask for help and follow the officer right to
the hospital.

When he got there, he found his son Tim in intensive
care with a serious head injury. He was told by the medic
helicopter crew that "the other one is alive," so Conrad,
of course, assumed that meant Rick. He didn't know Rick's
roommate had been asleep in the backseat of the car and
was the "alive one" who had escaped with only a scratch.

Within moments every parent's worst nightmare came
true.

"The nurse kept telling me, 'You've got to realize your son is dead,'" Conrad recalls. "She could tell I was in shock.

"I started calling people [on the phone] and telling them 'Rick's dead,' but there was no feeling in my voice. A few hours later it finally hit me, and I cried and cried."

The next day my husband and I got the call about the boys' accident from a member of the Songsters' church, where my husband had first been a pastor. We live only a couple of hours from Bethesda, so we dropped everything and drove down to the hospital where Rick had been pronounced dead and Tim was fighting for his life. Dot already had arrived with their eldest son, Jeff, his wife, and Tim's girlfriend.

They were all together in a private lounge at the hospital when we walked in. We hadn't called ahead, so our arrival was completely unexpected. But one look at their faces told us it was the best decision we could have made.

We hugged and sobbed together for what seemed a very long time. We said nothing profound, but I could tell they all were drawing new strength from us to face the next hour. We prayed with them and with Tim. The agony on their faces was so hard to watch as they struggled to grieve for one son and yet give hope to another.

We drove back down to the hospital two days later, and my husband led a beautiful memorial service for Rick at the chapel in Bethesda Naval Hospital (where Tim had been transferred). Many of Rick's brand-new, yet incredibly supportive, IBM colleagues attended.

About two weeks later when Tim was healed enough to go home, the family had another service to celebrate Rick's short life.

Rick has been gone for more than seventeen years as I write this, but when I chatted with the Songsters in their living room not long ago, the tears flowed freely again for all of us.

"You never get over it," Conrad says. "I still can cry in a second. A lot of times I sit in church and bawl," he admits. "A certain hymn or something just does it, but I'm not ashamed to say that happens."

Conrad's intense grief is not surprising, as there is something so unnatural and unnerving about outliving your child.

Author and pastor Dan Hans, who lost his three-year-old daughter to a brain tumor, says, "To lose a parent is to lose your past; to lose a spouse or close friend is to lose your present; and to lose a child is to lose your future."[1] Each death shakes a little different part of your world.

Conrad acknowledges that he still thinks about how his future has been changed without having Rick in his world.

"Sometimes I think about him and I wonder if he'd be married now and if he'd have kids and what they'd be

---

1. Daniel T. Hans, *When a Child Dies* (Matthews, NC: Desert Ministries, 1998), 1.

like," he says, wiping a tear from his cheek. "Somebody once told me that 'God needed another flower in Heaven,' but that stuff just doesn't cut it for me.

"I remember coming to the funeral home and someone saying, 'I know just how you feel,'" he recalls. "That's a bunch of baloney. People don't know just how you feel. All I wanted was someone to listen to me and not tell me how I felt."

While well-meaning but misguided comments from friends did not help the couple get through their grief, other things did. They met with a grief counselor and talked about the different ways people grieve. Acknowledging each other's unique personalities and diverse coping techniques helped them have more realistic expectations of themselves and each other. The outpouring of love and support from family and friends, especially their church family, continually picked them up when they needed it most.

"We still have a big box of [sympathy] cards from people," Conrad says. "I don't think we'll ever get rid of those."

At first the couple really struggled with their faith in God and why the accident happened.

"You rationalize it from a human perspective and think that God's punishing you for something," Conrad says. "But through talking with friends, reading Scripture, and praying, you learn that God doesn't do that."

It took many long months of searching and praying, but the couple says they have reconciled the two seemingly contradictory notions: that God loves them and yet didn't spare Rick's life.

"I still don't know why God allowed it to happen," Dot says. "But I'm not mad anymore."

Not only did their anger at God cease, but they also began to see that in a strange, supernatural way, God actually was the One who was supplying what they needed to get through each day, each hour, and each minute.

"We had the strength from God to get through," Conrad explains. "We couldn't do it on our own, but He could do it through us."

Bereavement counselor Robert Zucker explains that "healing from a deep loss is *not* about 'recovery' and returning to 'the way things were.'" Rather, it's about "allowing ourselves to keep on changing and becoming, amidst the pain."[2]

But we don't usually want to change and grow, do we? I know that a few months after Rick's death when I was diagnosed with cancer and given a 40 percent chance to survive, I desperately wanted to turn the clock back to those much happier B.C. (Before Cancer) days. Instead I went through surgery, six months of extremely difficult chemotherapy, the daily fear that I wouldn't see my daughters grow up (they were eight, ten, and twelve at the time),

2. "What I've Learned from Grief," *CareNotes* (St. Meinrad, IN: Abbey Press, 2001).

and the agony of knowing my husband was wondering if he would bury another wife. (He lost his first wife to ALS/ Lou Gehrig's disease when they were newlyweds.)

The last thing I wanted to do was change or grow, but turning back the clock was not an option. Every time I attend yet another funeral for a dear friend or family member, I know there is only one change I want: to have him or her back in my life.

But I can't do that any more than you can bring back your loved ones. They are gone, and we are never going to change that fact. Now we are faced with the choice of whether to allow God to change and teach us even in the midst of our pain.

> *"Come to me, all of you who are weary and carry heavy burdens, and I will give you rest. Take my yoke upon you. Let me teach you, because I am humble and gentle at heart, and you will find rest for your souls."*
> JESUS SPEAKING IN MATTHEW 11:28-29

Rest for your souls . . . doesn't that sound great? It is possible, you know. No matter what you've faced or what you still are facing, Jesus can give you rest for your weary soul.

Throughout this book you will meet dozens of grievers who are in the process of finding the strength to carry on.

> *My eyes are straining to see your promises come true. When will you comfort me?* PSALM 119:82

Others have been grieving for years and know first-hand that He is able.

Your promise revives me; it comforts me in all my troubles. PSALM 119:50

Their stories have striking similarities as well as diverse details. Yet a common thread runs through each story line: the realization that we don't *get over* grief. As sociologist and author Dr. Robert S. Weiss observes about those who have lived with long-standing loss: "You don't really get over it; you get used to it."[3]

The prophet Jeremiah writes of his own suffering and homelessness: "I will never forget this awful time, as I grieve over my loss."[4]

When the Jewish patriarch Jacob thought his son Joseph was dead, as Genesis 37:34-35 tells us, "He mourned deeply for his son for a long time. His family all tried to comfort him, but he refused to be comforted. 'I will go to my grave mourning for my son,' he would say, and then he would weep."

It is *not* your goal to get over your grief. How would you do that, anyway? Stop thinking about your loved one? Never cry for your loss? Live as if nothing has changed?

3. Robert S. Weiss, e-mail exchange with author, May 2, 2008.
4. Lamentations 3:20

Those are all ridiculous notions. Rebecca Rice, a therapist I know, says that grief is *not* resolved when we stop thinking about our loss. Instead, she says, a "major sign of grief resolution involves being able to think about the loss realistically, without experiencing an overwhelming sense of despair."[5]

Isn't that what your weary soul would like? To be able to think about your loved one's life—however brief or long—and yet not feel the intense pain?

My prayer is that God will use the words in this book to help you do just that. To let go of the feelings that need to be released without letting go of the love you never want to lose. I pray that other grievers' stories will encourage you that it won't always hurt as much or as deeply as it does right now.

"It's not that I don't think about Rick every day; I still do," Conrad acknowledges. "It just doesn't hurt so much every day."

Counselors Dr. Henry Cloud and Dr. John Townsend say that people need two things in order to grieve: love, which involves comfort and support; and structure, which involves time and space for grieving.[6] It is my prayer that this book will give you both.

---

5. Rebecca K. H. Rice, "A Word to Those Who Mourn . . ." (Lebanon, PA: Pennsylvania Counseling Services, n.d.).
6. Henry Cloud and John Townsend, *How People Grow* (Grand Rapids: Zondervan, 2001), 233.

When they walk through the Valley of Weeping, it will become a place of refreshing springs. Psalm 84:6

And as you walk through your personal Valley of Weeping, please remember you are walking *through* it—it is not your final destination. God has something else in store for you as He meets you in your grief.

I believe you are going to discover two things in this valley: You are much stronger than you think . . . and God is much greater than you think.

TAKE COMFORT: You'll never get over your loss, but you can get through it.

3

FINDING A FRIEND WHO UNDERSTANDS

My friends Donna and Jackie have become close friends
in a way they never would have wanted: as new widows
both facing a cancer diagnosis themselves.

The similarities in their stories are uncanny, right
down to the fact that they live a block away from each
other. Yet they never met until they both showed up at
a cancer workshop I was leading. I'm quite certain that
God brought us all together so He could show them just
how much He cares for the brokenhearted.

Donna's world was shaken first. In March 2003 her husband of thirty-nine years dropped dead of a heart attack
at the age of sixty.

"It was a Saturday morning and Frank was in the
garage," Donna recalls. "My four-year-old grand-
daughter, Shelby, opened the garage door and saw him

sitting on the bench. She said, 'Mom-Mom, come and look at Pop.'

"To this day I don't actually remember walking or running to him," Donna says. "But when I got to him, I could see he was already gone, and I just started screaming."

Her son Wayne came running from inside the house to his dad's side, but his attempts at CPR were unsuccessful. When the ambulance crew arrived shortly, they could not bring him back either.

At fifty-seven, Donna was a widow.

But that was only the beginning of the events that would shake her world. A chest X-ray that had been taken after a recent minor car accident had shown a shadow on one of her lungs. Further tests revealed a tumor the size of a lemon.

"Frank passed away before I got the official diagnosis, but three weeks later I found out I had [inoperable] lung cancer," she recalls.

Donna says her sons wanted her to quickly find an oncologist and start treatment, but her answer was "Why bother?"

"I was so depressed and anxious that I didn't really care if I got the cancer treated or not," she explains. "I would have to say I was a real basket case. I was trying to grieve, but with cancer, too, I didn't know how to do it all."

Thankfully Donna did find an oncologist, who practices in our building and who then referred her to me. I met Donna about two months after Frank's death, and in short course we became good friends, talking and praying often. I invited her to an American Cancer Society workshop for newly diagnosed patients, and that's where she met Jackie in the fall of 2005.

Jackie's world started to crash when her husband, Donald, sixty-one, was diagnosed with inoperable stomach cancer in December 2004 and a medical center physician announced he had six months to live. I met the couple a month later when he became a patient of Marc's, receiving biweekly chemotherapy.

Donald's cancer never responded well to the treatments, and he began going downhill fairly quickly. Then in June their difficult journey hit another low: Jackie was diagnosed with breast cancer at the age of sixty.

"I hated to go home and tell him," she recalls. "But he knew right away as soon as I came in the door."

She had surgery and was making plans to start radiation treatments when, eight months after his own diagnosis, Donald passed away.

"I didn't even cry right away 'cause everybody was there and I was the one to protect everybody," Jackie explains. "After they all left, except my sister, I went back to the bed he died in and lay down right on his side of the bed and cried myself to sleep. It was the most awful thing of my life.

"Donny had retired just two months before he got

cancer, and we had all these plans to go here and there," Jackie recalls. "We had plans to go to Florida and to go out West."

Despite the heartbreak of those unfulfilled dreams, Jackie soon discovered God would not leave her alone in her grief.

His plan had started to unfold a few months before when He drew Jackie and Donald to our evening Cancer Prayer Support Group meetings, where they experienced His love from fellow strugglers. A desire to walk with God was planted in their hearts.

"Every time we'd come home from a meeting, we'd talk about things, and I'd say, 'We should go to church sometime,' and he'd say, 'Not yet,'" Jackie recalls.

My husband and I even visited with them in their backyard one day because I was afraid by the time Donald was "ready" he might not be physically well enough to make it to our service.

Neither Donald nor Jackie had been to worship regularly for about thirty years. But on a warm Sunday morning in August 2005, I was thrilled when I saw Donald's wheelchair roll through our church's front doors. I already had made room for it in the back row "just in case" he ever came.

Jackie was working that day, so Donald came with their youngest daughter, Holly. Afterward he told me he really liked being there and would be back the next week.

He made it only one more time, but he and I had

some wonderful talks and prayers together at his home. I could see he had found a love for God.

Just two weeks after his first visit to our church, he passed away.

"We planned on coming that [last] Sunday, but he had fallen on Saturday and just wasn't strong enough," Jackie recalls.

Still she hadn't expected him to die that day. He had spent the whole day sitting in his living room with the hospice chaplain, Scott, watching a NASCAR race.

"Scott stayed until 7 p.m., and when he left, he said a prayer with him," Jackie remembers.

Donald passed away later that night. Pastor Scott led his funeral a few days later, and the very next Sunday Jackie was back in worship with some of her family members.

She's rarely missed a Sunday in the more than two years since. Three of her four grown children now worship somewhere regularly (two with her at our church). Eight of her grandkids, her six great-grandkids, and a handful of her nieces and nephews usually attend with her. Last year she was baptized and shared with our congregation how her spiritual life has changed since her husband's diagnosis and death.

"I always believed in God, but I didn't take time for God before," Jackie explains. "God helped me get back to where I needed to be."

And that change of priorities is what led Jackie to become part of God's plan in Donna's life.

"We became friends right from the beginning," Jackie

recalls. "We really understood each other. We talked to each other once or twice a week, so I invited her to church."

I had been inviting Donna to church for about two years with no results. I knew she had faith but had allowed herself to wander away from God's family and had no church home. Yet she readily accepted Jackie's invitation, and her lukewarm faith soon grew warm and strong.

"It took me a while to love the Lord like I should have been all along," Donna confesses.

"I love being at church now," she adds. Donna has become active in our church's women's ministry, as well as both my grief and cancer support groups.

When I ask her what words of wisdom she has for grievers, she quickly responds: "Make sure the Lord is by your side—either connect with Him or reconnect with Him."

And that is how two brokenhearted widows each found a friend who shared her special grief and encountered a God who understands their pain.

When we honestly ask ourselves which persons in our lives mean the most to us, we often find that it is those who, instead of giving much advice, solutions, or cures, have chosen rather to share our pain and touch our wounds with a gentle and tender hand. The friend who can be silent with us in a moment of despair or confusion, who can stay with us in an hour of grief and bereavement, who can tolerate not-knowing, not-curing, not-healing, and face with us the reality of our powerlessness, that is the friend who cares.[1]

As I write this chapter, it has been more than five years since Donna was diagnosed with inoperable, incurable non-small cell lung cancer. She has been in and out of remissions and treatment. More than two years ago the cancer spread to her brain, but she was able to have a specialized laser procedure to remove the spot and keep it away until a very recent recurrence. Following a second brain surgery, she feels well again and still looks beautiful. Every time I see her, she tells me how good God has been to her in these past five years battling cancer without her husband at her side.

"I'm at peace," she often says, and the look in her eyes tells me she really is. Meanwhile, Jackie is cancer free and continues hormone treatment to help prevent a recurrence.

And do they both still miss their husbands and struggle every day with their absence? Of course they do. Their worlds have been shaken, but because they both have a spiritual foundation and believe God's Word is a trustworthy compass in their grief-storms, *they* have not fallen apart.

---

1. Henri Nouwen, *The Dance of Life: Weaving Sorrows and Blessings into One Joyful Step*, ed. Michael Ford (Notre Dame, IN: Ave Maria Press, 2006), 170.

*I know the LORD is always with me. I will not be shaken,
for he is right beside me.* PSALM 16:8

*He alone is my rock and my salvation, my fortress where
I will never be shaken.* PSALM 62:2

*God is our refuge and strength,
    always ready to help in times of trouble.
So we will not fear when earthquakes come
    and the mountains crumble into the sea.* PSALM 46:1-2

Both women have learned that, contrary to the beautiful Bette Midler song, God is *not* watching them from a distance. Instead, He is very near, feeling their pain and even their grief.

The Jewish prophet Isaiah described the coming Messiah as one who "was despised and rejected—a man of sorrows, acquainted with deepest grief" (Isaiah 53:3). Jesus truly does understand how you feel. He understands partly because He is God and therefore knows everything. But He understands, not just from an intellectual perspective, but also from His own life experience.

Dorothy Sayers, the early twentieth-century British novelist and medieval scholar, describes how and why God understands our feelings.

For whatever reason God chose to make man as he is—limited and suffering and subject to sorrows and death—He had the honesty and the courage to take

His own medicine. Whatever game He is playing with His creation, He has kept His own rules and played fair. . . . He has Himself gone through the whole of human experience, from the trivial irritations of family life and the cramping restrictions of hard work and lack of money to the worst horrors of pain and humiliation, defeat, despair, and death.[2]

Can you imagine worshiping a God who is immune to pain? What if He never felt a slap, never knew the pang of betrayal, never experienced misery with no relief in sight? Such a God could never sympathize with our weaknesses or understand our pain. But because God "played" by the same rules we must play by (Rule no. 1: Life's not fair), He clearly understands what you and I feel. He was willing to endure agonizing pain and death on our behalf. And the best part is that He not only understands our sorrow, He has the power to do something about it.

The prophet Isaiah foretold that the Messiah would be sent by God "to comfort the brokenhearted."[3] At the Sermon on the Mount, Jesus told his listeners, "God blesses those who mourn, for they will be comforted."[4]

Jesus understands what it's like for your world to be shaken because His world was shaken too. He knows how to comfort you.

2. Dorothy L. Sayers, *Christian Letters to a Post-Christian World*, ed. Roderick Jellema (Grand Rapids: Eerdmans, 1969), 14.
3. Isaiah 61:1
4. Matthew 5:4

The Sovereign LORD has given me his words of wisdom, so that I know how to comfort the weary. ISAIAH 50:4

For I have given rest to the weary and joy to the sorrowing. JEREMIAH 31:25

For the LORD has comforted his people and will have compassion on them in their suffering. ISAIAH 49:13

Are you brokenhearted today? Are you weary of the storm of grief around you? Are you wondering how to pick up and put back together the shattered pieces of your world? If so, won't you pray and ask God to show you the comfort He promises to those who grieve? I can't promise you exactly how and when His answer will come, but I know why it will—because He loves you. Pure and simple. The almighty God of the universe loves you. As author Max Lucado writes: "If God had a refrigerator, your picture would be on it. If he had a wallet, your photo would be in it. He sends you flowers every spring and a sunrise every morning. Whenever you want to talk, he'll listen."[5]

Donna and Jackie recognize that God orchestrated their meeting—a sure sign of His care for them. Tell God today that you also need to be able to *feel* His love for you. Ask Him to show you in some way—perhaps a way that might make sense only to you—that He cares. If you have a trusted friend with faith, ask him or her to

5. *A Gentle Thunder* (Nashville: W Publishing, 1995), 122.

pray this for you too. And if you don't know anyone to ask or have a hard time praying for yourself, don't worry; just believe—because I've already been praying for you.

> *The Spirit of the Sovereign LORD is upon me. . . .*
> *He has sent me to comfort the brokenhearted. . . .*
> *He has sent me to tell those who mourn*
>   *that the time of the LORD's favor has come.*
> ISAIAH PROPHESYING ABOUT THE COMING MESSIAH, JESUS,
>   IN ISAIAH 61:1-2

> *With this news, strengthen those who have tired hands,*
>   *and encourage those who have weak knees.*
> *Say to those with fearful hearts,*
>   *"Be strong, and do not fear,*
> *for your God is coming to destroy your enemies.*
>   *He is coming to save you."* ISAIAH 35:3-4

TAKE COMFORT: God specializes in blessing those who mourn.

4

Preserving a Memory
No One Can Steal

I wish you could attend one of our Grief Prayer Support Group meetings. We gather monthly in a small conference room and often have to bring in extra chairs. We drink coffee and tea and enjoy everything from warm Krispy Kreme donuts to angel food cake with fresh strawberries made by one of the widowers who follows his wife's favorite recipe.

As I've already mentioned, I always start out the meeting with jokes because when your world is shaken there's usually not much to laugh or even smile about. If there are first-timers at our meeting, I might begin by saying: "I know grief is not funny, but I believe the Bible when it says that laughter is good medicine.[1] So I'm going to share a few jokes today. You don't have to laugh if you don't want to. But you may find that just a little smile will appear on your face and you'll feel a little more alive because this is a safe place to both cry and laugh."

---

1. See Proverbs 17:22

The group regulars have come to look forward to my dumb jokes (I especially love puns), but I must admit I still get nervous when someone who recently suffered a loss arrives for the first time. This happened a couple of weeks ago when a mother came who had just buried her daughter the month before. Her daughter Deb was a beautiful woman, only forty-two years old. Deb had been raising her two children by herself after her husband walked out on her when he learned she had a recurrence of cancer. For a moment that morning, I considered skipping the jokes because I knew Kathy was not in a laughing mood.

But instead, I said a quick, silent prayer and shared my jokes. To my amazement the grieving mother smiled weakly at every punch line. At the end of the meeting, she hugged me and thanked me for our time together. I knew a tiny bit of healing had taken place in her broken heart, because I believe that when grievers laugh together, they are reminded that they can let go of the intense pain without betraying the memory of their loved one. We need to be reminded that just because we laugh, it doesn't mean we don't still grieve our loved ones.

King Solomon said it well:

> *For everything there is a season,*
> *a time for every activity under heaven. . . .*
> *A time to cry and a time to laugh.*
> *A time to grieve and a time to dance.* Ecclesiastes 3:1, 4

"What this group has taught me is how to laugh again," says Jim, who joined our little "grieving gang" shortly after he lost Jane, his wife of fifty-eight years. "I'm sure the hurt will never go away because of the void in my life, but it does feel good to laugh again."

While it was wonderful that Jim and Jane had almost six decades together as a couple, that longevity of enjoying one another's company makes the loneliness that much fiercer now.

There's probably something about your grief-storm that makes life without your loved one especially difficult. It seems as if all the grievers in my group have unique twists to their situations, which magnifies their mourning. There is:

- Charlie B., who feels the loneliness more than many do because he has no children or grandchildren to keep him company after losing Mary, his beloved wife of forty-five years
- Mike, whose fifty-nine-year-old wife, Annie, was diagnosed with cancer so late, she came home from the hospital on hospice and died within two months
- Rita, who is coping with a double measure of grief after losing her husband, Francis, and then her mentally challenged adult son, Tom, exactly a week later
- Linda, whose husband, Mike, seemed to be responding well to his treatments but unexpectedly died

in bed one night only a few hours after a great day
that included going out to dinner and mowing the
yard

- Ralph, whose wife, Carol, passed away the day before
their son's wedding
- Peg, who is plagued with guilt that she should have
done more to alleviate her husband's suffering
- Al, who lost his wife and adult daughter to cancer and
is now fighting the disease himself
- Charlie O., who is forced to face life not only without his wife but also childless and without parents
or siblings
- Sally, who is still frustrated with financial and insur-
ance wrangling several months after losing her husband, Ric, who always shared in these matters during
their forty-three years of marriage
- Jeanette, whose husband, Bob, was diagnosed on a
Thursday and passed away the next Tuesday
- Bill, who at ninety-one has outlived two wives, the
second one of whom was twenty-one years his junior
and married him when he was eighty-eight!

Do any of their situations remind you of your own
personal pain? There probably are some similarities,
but you could add your own details that make your
grief unique.

> *Each heart knows its own bitterness, and no one else can
> fully share its joy.* PROVERBS 14:10

I love that proverb. When I apply it to grievers, it tells me that no earthly person really can know the depth of your bitter grief, but at the same time no one else fully shares the joy you have in your heart as you recall your wonderful memories of your loved one. The healing in your heart starts, I believe, when you can begin to look past the bitter death of your loved one and begin to celebrate his or her joyful life.

Mike, an electrical engineer in our group, says he has been "trying to make that mental shift" in the past year since he lost his wife, Annie, so suddenly.

"I feel that it is the way my wife died that has made it so hard on me," Mike says. "I hope the day will come when I stop thinking about taking care of her while she was dying and start to remember the love, joy, and happiness we had before she got cancer."

I admire Mike's painful honesty when he talks about his grief at our group. I've watched him try to sort through the years of memories—doing his best to hang on to the beautiful ones and hoping to release the painful ones.

"I have a notebook, and I'm starting to write about all the wonderful things we did in life," he says.

Mike and Annie had a home in the woods, and both shared an affinity for nature and the changing seasons, which inspired her beautiful watercolor paintings. So Mike built an outdoor rock memorial for Annie inside the shade garden they had made together. He finds solace when he visits it and knows his wife would have loved it too.

"I want to let go of the pain and the sorrow, not the love and the memories," he adds. "There are times I wish I could forget about her death, but that would mean I'd have to forget about her."

Death leaves a heartache no one can heal; love leaves a memory no one can steal.

From a headstone in Ireland

Aren't you thankful no one can steal your precious memories of your loved one? Several participants in my grief group either have created tangible reminders of their precious memories or have had others do so for them. Linda's sister-in-law made her a teddy bear out of one of her husband's favorite Penn State shirts—replete with a little Nittany Lion mascot on the paw.

"Mike would have loved it," Linda says. "Sometimes I put a little of his aftershave on it, and I sit and hold it because it smells just like him."

Another widow took some of her husband's vast T-shirt "collection" to a friend who cut the treasured tops into squares for a patchwork quilt. She loves covering up in it and feeling her husband's presence in a special way.

When my maternal grandfather died, my aunt Sherry cut up his old, black police department shirts and made little vests from them. Each vest had a shiny, gold "PD" button sewn on it and a police insignia patch stitched to it. All nine of his adult children got a vest-wearing teddy bear, which still reminds them of the years their dad proudly served in the police department.

My friend Connie, whose story I'll tell in detail later, has a lovely quilt made from her deceased husband's work shirts and jeans. It's a beautiful mosaic of riveted pockets, frayed cuffs, worn cotton, and faded denim, which allows Connie to wrap up in the unending warmth of his love for her.

Charlie B. leaves out his wife's Christmas angel collection all year because he knows how much she cherished each figurine, and they are a wonderful reminder to him of her beauty. And my friend Gigi, whom you'll also meet later, created a "little wall to honor my dad" filled with framed photos from the many pictures he enjoyed taking over the years.

My friend Barry is probably one of the last people I would expect to create a healing memory of his wife, Barbara. He's a great guy, but he has a tough-guy persona. I'll tell you more about Barry and his incredible wife in a later chapter, but for now I just want to share with you one of the ways he helped himself and his family move past Barb's death to celebrate her life—away from bitterness and toward joy.

"I knew [the first] Christmas was going to be hard," Barry says.

All four grown kids would be home with Barry, three

with spouses and one with a little baby. Barb's folks and siblings would be there too. But the wife/mother/ grandmother/daughter/sister/aunt who loved them all so deeply would not.

However, Barry wanted to make sure Barb *was* "there" that day, so he asked a friend with computer skills to help produce a CD with a slideshow presentation of Barb's life. The photos included such things as their college days, her field hockey games, their wedding thirty-four years before, and their kids' growing-up years and college graduations. The images were accompanied by music, beginning with Kenny Rogers singing "Through the Years," followed by Barbra Streisand's poignant tune "Memories" and Josh Groban's "You Raise Me Up." At the end, the screen settled on one last picture of Barb with her one-month-old grandson, Braden, just before her death in February. (When I watched the recording later, I made it to Kenny Rogers singing, "You're the love of my life, you're my lady" before I was reduced to a puddle.)

Barry also wrote a letter to each family member, including Barb's extended family, and tucked it in with the CDs.

"It was really hard to do, but God just put it on my heart to do it," he explains.

Barry's family sat mesmerized watching the thirty-minute tribute that Christmas Eve, and dry eyes were hard to find. As they left that evening, the guests clutched their own precious copies.

Barry says he still listens to the CD soundtrack in the

car even though it is "torture" sometimes to realize how much he misses his wife.

He is right that grief can be torture. It is hard work. It's tempting to try to numb our feelings through things like pills, alcohol, food, TV, or even busyness. But when the numbness wears off, the pain still will be there. It's tough for Barry and others who force themselves to do the hard work of grieving, because they must face things they really don't want to face and allow themselves to feel things they'd really rather not feel. But the hard work leads to healing.

Time doesn't heal all things; it's what we do with the time that heals.

Dot and Conrad, whom you met in the second chapter, both found that the time they spent with their recovering son, Tim, helped them grieve the loss of their son Rick.

"I think God let us heal some by taking care of Tim in those weeks after the accident," Dot says.

When Tim had recovered enough to return to the Air Force Academy, Conrad spent time every day writing a short note to him with a verse of Scripture included. By his graduation, Tim had received more than nine hundred notes.

"Tim said he was really helped in his grief by my sending the letters and Scriptures to him," Conrad says. "As I recall, it also gave me a mission and made me get through the immediate grief."

What a beautiful way to use time wisely to heal.

One of the things I'd like to suggest you do with your time is this: learn to trust God in a deeper way.

We often hear the phrase "Let go and let God," and it can seem rather trite. What does it mean, anyway? Drop everything and God will pick it up? Sit back and do nothing while God takes care of everything?

For grievers, I believe it means to trust God as you begin to let go of the intense pain and start to let God fill the emptiness with Himself.

> *I will never forget this awful time,*
> *   as I grieve over my loss.*
> *Yet I still dare to hope*
> *   when I remember this:*
>
> *The faithful love of the LORD never ends!*
> *   His mercies never cease.*
> *Great is his faithfulness;*
> *   his mercies begin afresh each morning.*
> LAMENTATIONS 3:20-23

Begin to let go of the painful memories surrounding your loved one's death and let God help you celebrate his or her life.

> *Weeping may last through the night, but joy comes with the morning.* PSALM 30:5

Begin to let go of the plans you had and let God show you His plan for you.

> *"For I know the plans I have for you," says the* LORD. *"They are plans for good and not for disaster, to give you a future and a hope."* JEREMIAH 29:11

I wish I could include a CD with this book. It would feature "Spirit Song," a beautiful song about trusting Jesus enough to "let Him have those things that hold you." If you know the song, sing along to yourself (or out loud if you're not in a public place!). If you don't, perhaps you can listen to the song online or just read the words now and let them sink deeply into your heart.

> *O let the Son of God enfold you*
> *With His Spirit and His love*
> *Let Him fill your heart and satisfy your soul*
> *O let Him have those things that hold you*
> *And His Spirit like a dove*
> *Will descend upon your life*
> *And make you whole*
>
> *(chorus)*
> *Jesus, O Jesus, come and fill your lambs*
> *Jesus, O Jesus, come and fill your lambs*
>
> *O come and sing this song with gladness*
> *As your hearts are filled with joy*
> *Lift your hands in sweet surrender*
> *To His name*

O give Him all your tears and sadness
Give Him all your years of pain
And you'll enter into life
In Jesus' name[2]

TAKE COMFORT: Let go of the emptiness and let God fill it with Himself.

2. John Wimber, "Spirit Song," copyright ©1979 Mercy/Vineyard Publishing (ASCAP). Administered in North America by Music Services o/b/o Vineyard Music USA. All rights reserved. Used by permission.

5

Being Held Up

If you want to start a lively discussion sometime, just
ask a roomful of grievers whether anyone has made an
insensitive remark to them since their loved ones died.
I guarantee you the recollections will be vivid, free
flowing, and still hurtful no matter how much time
has passed.

> "God wanted another flower in His garden."
> "At least you have other children."
> "God must have needed her more than you do."
> "At least he lived a long life."
> "You're young—you'll find someone else."
> "I thought you'd be over this by now."

I actually entertained the idea of writing a whole book
about stupid comments made to grievers but decided
that probably wouldn't be all that productive. I did,
however, discover there are plenty of Web sites and chat
rooms dedicated to just such inane remarks.

I once did begin an adult class on grief with the question: "Did anyone make any insensitive comments to you after your loved one's death?" An hour later I still was getting an earful, and after class people lined up to share more painful comments with me.

Eileen, a lovely, generous woman with a strong faith, recalled that after her husband died unexpectedly from cancer at the age of fifty-seven, a friend cheerfully announced to her: "God can be your husband now."

"I did not want God to be my husband and I told her so," Eileen said with a firmness I hadn't expected from her.

Charlie B. from my support group recalled that about six months after his wife, Mary, died, he was telling a relative how much he missed her, and the relative responded: "You have to get over that." Then a couple of years later he ran into a former coworker at Wal-Mart who commented: "I thought you would have a new honey by now."

"People know that I miss her, but they don't understand the depth of my feelings," Charlie said. "On the outside I seem to be normal. But deep in my heart there are no words to describe the awful pain of not having her with me."

I remember when I miscarried our first baby at three months gestation—on Mother's Day of all days. That night a nurse came by my hospital room and told me: "You're young—you'll have other children."

While her words were logical (and eventually did come true), they did not comfort me: I didn't want a "replacement" baby—I wanted the child I already loved. I needed to grieve the baby I would hold only in my heart and never in my arms.

Through the years as I've heard my share of insensitive remarks, I've tried to remind myself that most people mean well and just don't know what to say. I realize I need to "hear" their hearts and not just their words.

One of the most insensitive remarks I ever heard came out after that same adult class with Eileen. A gentleman in his seventies whom I'll call Fred stayed after class to privately share his "horror" story with me.

He told me his three-year-old son had been tragically killed in an accident more than thirty years before. He spoke of the details as if it were yesterday.

His son was next door playing with the neighbor boy when a heavy storm window, which was leaning against the house, fell on him and killed him instantly. Fred was first on the scene and had to lift the window from his little son's lifeless body.

According to Fred, the neighbor was "a Christian and a Bible-believing man." One can only imagine how that man must have felt about such an accident occurring on his property—perhaps guilty for not putting away the storm windows. But what he said to Fred was unthinkable.

"He told me, 'I guess you'll have to thank us for putting your son in Heaven,'" Fred recalled.

I made no attempt to hide my shock as I asked him how in the world he responded to that.

"I thought for a moment and then I said, 'I know my son's in Heaven, but I don't thank you for that—I thank Jesus Christ. And I hope I never take a drink again because if I do, I might be sending you to Heaven!'"

> *I have heard all this before.*
> *What miserable comforters you are!*
> *Won't you ever stop blowing hot air?*
> *What makes you keep on talking?*
> *I could say the same things if you were in my place.*
> *I could spout off criticism and shake my head at you.*
> *But if it were me, I would encourage you.*
> *I would try to take away your grief. . . .*
> *How can your empty clichés comfort me?* Job 16:2-5; 21:34

People talk about having "the patience of Job" because he probably suffered more grief than any other person on the face of the earth. Job was a prosperous farmer who lost all his children, his servants, his home, and his livestock. Then to add insult to injury, he was afflicted with painful sores all over his body.

Three of his friends, Eliphaz, Bildad, and Zophar (great names if you ever have triplets in your family), talked to him about the "reasons" for his tragedies. They told Job his sin had caused his suffering, despite the fact that they knew Job was a righteous man. Finally Job had enough of their insensitive remarks and responded by calling them "miserable comforters."

But the interesting thing is that his three friends, E, B, and Z, didn't start out as miserable comforters—in fact they first responded just the way I think most of us would want our comforters to. Back up to Job chapter 2 and you'll see what I mean.

> *When three of Job's friends heard of the tragedy he had suffered, they got together and traveled from their homes to comfort and console him. Their names were Eliphaz the Temanite, Bildad the Shuhite, and Zophar the Naamathite. When they saw Job from a distance, they scarcely recognized him. Wailing loudly, they tore their robes and threw dust into the air over their heads to show their grief. Then they sat on the ground with him for seven days and nights. No one said a word to Job, for they saw that his suffering was too great for words.* JOB 2:11-13*

They saw that his suffering was too great for words so they simply sat quietly with him for a week feeling his pain. Don't you wish some of your friends, relatives, and coworkers realized that about your suffering? That it's too great for words? That no explanation they offer will fix things? Then they would be real comforters.

Now I realize I'm writing a book of *words*. But I have no illusion that these words are going to explain your suffering or "fix" anything for you. However, I do have faith that our all-powerful God can supernaturally take my words—and especially His Word—and use them to comfort you. He'll be your comfort, not I.

That being said, I also know that people are often the *means* God uses to deliver His comfort. Right now my laptop is plugged into the wall socket. The power cord is the means by which the computer is getting its power, but it's not the source. God is the source of all comfort, but people often are the means of delivering that comfort.

That's why it's so crucial for you to resist the urge to go it alone with your grief. And that's why I pray you find good comforters who will deliver God's consolation to you.

That's exactly what has happened to my good friend Charlie O. (Members of our grief group call him that to distinguish him from Charlie B.)

Charlie O. is by nature a loner. He's a quiet, introverted, hardworking factory guy who would rather stay home and watch a NASCAR race on his big-screen TV than attend a lively party somewhere. He has few living relatives—he was an only child and both his parents are dead. He and his wife, Vicki, had no children together.

I knew Vicki for about two years before she died. I met her in 2002 in the hospital just after she found out her rare cancer had returned following a four-year remission. She was in many ways the opposite of her husband. She was outgoing and loved to talk, even to strangers. She was a real animal lover and bred adorable

Chihuahuas and beautiful songbirds. We quickly became good friends. Though initially she told me her spiritual faith was unimportant to her, soon she began attending my morning Cancer Prayer Support Group (and bringing delicious homemade cakes to each meeting).

God began working in Vicki's heart, healing past hurts that had caused her to leave faith behind for more than thirty years. In May 2003 she finally got up the courage to walk through the front doors of my church. As she did, she burst into tears from the emotion of coming to worship after so many decades. A week later at another Sunday morning service, she responded to an invitation from an eighty-six-year-old visiting preacher to "give your life to God because you belong to God." Exactly one year and one day later, she died.

When Vicki passed away, I had no hope that Charlie would draw close enough for God to comfort him in his grief. Except for once at Christmas, he had refused to come with his wife to worship. She often had asked him to attend, but he simply wasn't interested in spiritual matters. I figured that without her requests he would have no incentive to come at all.

So I was really shocked when Charlie came up to me after Vicki's memorial service at our church and told me he wanted to start coming to worship.

"I figured since she passed away and you were a good friend to Vicki and me, I'd start coming," Charlie later explained to me. "I thought that probably would be good for me."

Now, more than three years later, Charlie says that decision has been "very good" for him. On the Easter following Vicki's death, Charlie asked Jesus to forgive his sins and become the leader of his life. And then a few weeks later, quiet, introverted Charlie stepped completely out of his comfort zone as he stood before our congregation at his baptism and gave a tearful testimony of God's faithfulness to him during his grief-storm.

"My faith is growing more all the time," he says. "I'm still shy—I don't think that's ever going to change."

Charlie says he can't imagine how he would have faced widowerhood if he had not come to our Grief Prayer Support Group and our church. "The grief group and everyone at church is my family—you're all I've got," he explains. "I'm grateful for everything God and everybody has done for me."

And I'm so grateful God would work in Charlie's life despite my lack of faith that he would ever let God meet his grief.

Charlie has experienced what counselors Dr. Henry Cloud and Dr. John Townsend describe as the necessity of "a letting-down" and "a letting-go" in grief.

"[An] important reason people cannot grieve the way they need to is that they lack resources. In short, grief is a letting-down and a letting-go. And we cannot let down and let go if we are not being held up," they write. "If there is not enough love to sustain us, both inside and out, then we cannot let go of anything, even something bad."[1]

I have observed that many grievers need to let go of one thing: regrets.

A few people in my grief group say they have no regrets surrounding their loved ones' last days and weeks, but many others are riddled with guilt over things they feel they should or shouldn't have done.

"Did I do the right thing?"

"Could I have done something more?"

"Why didn't I make him go to the doctor sooner?"

"Is there something I could have done to prevent this?"

"Why didn't I tell her more often that I loved her?"

Once, as I listened to members of our group sharing these painful regrets, I was struck by something fascinating: everyone there was willing (and able) to say that the others had done enough for their loved ones, but few were willing (or able) to say that of themselves. Each was certain that all the other caregivers had "tried hard enough," "couldn't have done anything else," and "shouldn't feel guilty." But only a couple of them were willing to extend that same grace to themselves.

Do you have enough love inside (from God) and enough love outside (from friends and family) that you

1. Henry Cloud and John Townsend, *How People Grow* (Grand Rapids: Zondervan, 2001), 233.

can let down your emotions and let go of things like guilty regrets? Do you need to find someone who will help you feel God's comfort? It is possible, you know. It might be another griever with a situation similar to your own, like Donna and Jackie found in each other. Or it might be a congregation of believers who have a love for hurting people, as Charlie found in our church. Or it might be a counselor with faith who has expertise in tearing down the walls so God's light can shine on your darkness.

I don't know if you believe in Satan or not, but I do. He's not a cartoon character in a red suit with a pitchfork. The Bible says he is a personal force of evil who comes to "steal and kill and destroy."[2] I believe Satan wants to steal your joy, kill your desire to go on, and destroy your peace—and one of the best ways he can do that is to keep you isolated. As long as you are continually by yourself without real faith-filled comforters, he can keep you cut off from God's peace.

I believe he's also the one who wants to keep your mind filled with guilty regrets. The Bible calls him "the accuser" (Revelation 12:10). He loves to whisper half-truths in our ears, charging us with things we "should have" or "could have" done.

Won't you pray today and ask the Lord to guide you to true comforters: those who won't accuse you but will encourage you—people who will help you let go

---

2. John 10:10

of whatever you need to release to God? I believe He's already started that process by leading you to this book. Even if we never meet, I hope I can be a true comforter to you, helping you feel God's lavish love for the brokenhearted.

The Jewish apostle Paul, who preached the gospel to the Gentiles, describes how God once sent someone to encourage him when he was down and out.

> *When we arrived in Macedonia, there was no rest for us. We faced conflict from every direction, with battles on the outside and fear on the inside. But God, who encourages those who are discouraged, encouraged us by the arrival of Titus. His presence was a joy.* 2 CORINTHIANS 7:5-7

Never forget that we serve a God who "encourages those who are discouraged." When Paul "faced conflict from every direction," God sent his friend Titus at just the right time to fill him with joy. God knows exactly what you need to deal with today's discouragement. Ask Him to send a "Titus" (or two) to encourage you, and then wait to see His awesome answer.

> *I prayed to the LORD, and he answered me.*
> *He freed me from all my fears.*
> *Those who look to him for help will be radiant with joy;*
> *no shadow of shame will darken their faces.*
> *In my desperation I prayed, and the LORD listened;*
> *he saved me from all my troubles.* PSALM 34:4-6

I am counting on the LORD; *yes, I am counting on him.*
I have put my hope in his word. PSALM 130:5

TAKE COMFORT: God can comfort you through those who will
hold you up so you can let down and let go.

6

Comprehending the Incomprehensible

Whether we saw death coming or whether it struck unexpectedly, our minds struggle to comprehend the unthinkable: our loved one is really gone.

"My dad ate a bowl of ice cream, and ten minutes later he was gone," recalls one griever in my support group.

"I just left the room for a moment, and when I came back she was gone," says another.

"I keep thinking he's still going to come walking through the front door," laments a third.

"I feel like I should be tucking her in bed, but she's not there," whispers another.

No wonder our minds can't comprehend death; we can't imagine going on without our loved ones.

We long for just one more phone call.
We yearn for just one more smile.
We are desperate for just one more "I love you."

"People say to me, 'I bet it feels like your right arm has been cut off,' but it's a whole lot worse than that," observes my friend Connie, who was widowed at forty-seven. "It's more like my heart has been ripped out."

And even though my friend John's wife, Linda, was on hospice for more than a year and died peacefully in her sleep, he still says it feels "like a piece of me has been ripped away."

It's no exaggeration to say that since our loved ones died, a part of us is missing. If you are the mother or father of a child who died, that child literally was a part of you before birth. If you have lost a spouse, the two of you had became one, as the Bible says (Matthew 19:5), and could not be separated equally (just try to pull apart two pieces of glued corrugated cardboard without leaving bits of each stuck to the other half!). And if you have lost another close family member or dear friend, no doubt that person helped shape the person you are today. It seems unimaginable, but a part of us *has* died.

My friend David has faced the incomprehensible twice in the last eight of his seventy-five years of living.[1] First, his youngest son, Kevin, died of AIDS. Then his middle son, Alan, committed suicide. I talked to him recently, just a few months after Alan's death.

"These past months have been like a dream gone bad," David says. "My feelings have ranged from shock and disbelief to pain, anger, and guilt."

---

1. Names and a few details of David's story have been changed to protect his family's privacy.

David, a godly man of great faith who is a respected Bible teacher, is at a loss to understand how and why forty-nine-year-old Alan could do the unthinkable, leaving behind his wife and three children.

"Alan was a handsome, intelligent, free-spirited, fun-loving guy; a prankster with an extraordinary sense of humor who could make even the most orthodox [person] double over in laughter in a heartbeat," David recalls. "Alan was high voltage, fearless, and loved living life on the edge. He was into dirt bikes, hunting, catching rattlesnakes, and skydiving."

But in recent years Alan had become addicted to prescription painkillers he took to alleviate pain from several injuries and surgeries, David says. And on a cold winter day he left his Michigan home in deep despair and disappeared into some nearby woods, where he took his own life.

The days since Alan's death "have been most challenging to say the least," David admits. "Sudden waves of grief come rushing in from out of nowhere, twisting our souls with all kinds of emotional contortions."

And yet even as David's world has been terribly shaken again, God's supernatural strength is seeing him through.

"When we find ourselves in the deepest of despair, still *underneath* us are His everlasting arms," David explains. "As believers we are not immune to the tragedies of life— even when everything around us seems to collapse—but we never can be brought so low as to be beyond the reach of the Father's everlasting arms."

The eternal God is your refuge, and underneath are the everlasting arms. DEUTERONOMY 33:27, NIV

That's the verse that has given David great comfort in the aftermath of burying a third child. (Alan's twin sister, Allison, was stillborn, so only one of David's four children remains.) The verse reminds him, he says, of "God's enabling strength when we question whether we can traverse another day."

I felt a special bond with Barry and his beautiful wife, Barb, from the first time I met them after she was diagnosed with pancreatic cancer at age fifty-four. She was only a couple of years older than I, and their close-knit family, which included four grown kids who all loved God and sports, reminded me so much of my own family (we even each have a youngest daughter named Lindsey). It was easy—and painful—to imagine myself in Barb's situation as I watched her waver between hopeful optimism and sinking reality.

I especially wondered how Barry, a Division III football coach who prided himself on "mental toughness," would cope with Barb's inevitable death. I knew he was used to dishing out strength for others; but in the end watching his once-athletic wife ravaged by cancer and in unrelenting pain was beyond his own strength, Barry admits.

"There's no way I could have envisioned that I would have the strength to go through all that," he says. "God just gave it to me."

By His strength.

That was the mantra that saw Barry's family through Barb's devastating illness. Shortly after her diagnosis, Barb's younger brother Tommy bought silver bracelets for all the family members with the letters *BHS* engraved on the front. They stood for "by His strength." The bracelets were partly a Christian response to Lance Armstrong's "Live Strong" yellow plastic bracelets. But mostly they were a reminder to everyone that they could live strong through God's strength—even if they didn't have the strength within themselves. The initials *BHS* always reminded Barb's family of their heavenly Father and of their earthly family: Barbara Hall Streeter and Barry Howard Streeter.

> *But those who trust in the LORD will find new strength. They will soar high on wings like eagles.* Isaiah 40:31

That's the verse reference that was engraved on the back of the bracelets, and I watched Barb's entire family face her illness "by His strength," as their love, support, and prayers for each other poured out week after week. Barb lived eighteen months past her diagnosis—about three times the average for her kind of cancer—but her death was no less devastating to her family.

"It was about 3 a.m., and I knew her death was close,"

Barry recalls. "I woke everybody up, and they all came into the bedroom.

"God gave me the strength to lie down beside her in that bed knowing she was going to die any minute," he remembers as his eyes begin to tear. He recounts how he grabbed a Bible and read Isaiah 40:31 as well as Psalm 139, a favorite of Barb's.

"The kids were all there, and it was just such a spiritual thing," Barry recalls. "When she died, we knew she wasn't really there. Her body was just a shell, and she was with the Lord. It was just such an affirmation of what we believe."

Hundreds of athletes, friends, and family members attended Barb's memorial service at the college chapel. It was a continued affirmation of the family's great faith even as they sang the old hymn "It Is Well with My Soul."

Now I don't want to give you the impression that because of his great faith, Barry has it easy. Hardly. He is struggling with loneliness and sorrow and disbelief and questions just as you probably are.

When a friend called him on the first anniversary of Barb's death and asked if it was an especially hard day for him, Barry told him, "This day isn't really any worse than any other. It really stinks today, it was really stinking yesterday, and quite frankly it's going to really stink tomorrow without Barb."

"I'm heartbroken—that's exactly what I feel," he says now. "When you get married, you're one person, and part of me went with her."

I really appreciate Barry's openness and honesty. I share his words with you in hopes of encouraging you that you are not alone if you are struggling with grief in spite of having a strong faith. Trusting God does *not* protect us from trials, nor does it exempt us from anguish.

> *I am exhausted from crying for help;*
> *my throat is parched.*
> *My eyes are swollen with weeping,*
> *waiting for my God to help me.* Psalm 69:3

Those aren't words from an unbeliever but from the great Jewish king David, who was described as a man after God's own heart.

Author Joanie Yoder writes that in her second year of widowhood she was still struggling.

Morning after morning my prayer-life consisted of one daily sigh: "Lord, I shouldn't be struggling like this!" "And why not?" His still, small voice asked me from within one morning.

Then the answer came—unrecognized pride! Somehow I had thought that a person of my spiritual maturity should be beyond such struggle. What a ridiculous thought! I had never been a widow before and needed the freedom to be a true learner—even a struggling learner.[2]

Be gentle with yourself as you grieve. You're not getting a grade on your efforts; there are no Oscars for "Best Performance as a Griever." There is no easy, quick way out of a grief-storm.

But those who trust in the LORD will find new strength. They will soar high on wings like eagles. Isaiah 40:31

I've read that an eagle, like many other animals, can sense a storm before it arrives. So the eagle flies to a high spot and waits for the inevitable winds. When the storm hits, the eagle sets its wings so that the wind will pick it up and lift it above the storm. While the storm rages below, the eagle is soaring above it. The eagle does not escape the storm but simply rises on the winds to be lifted higher.

God has allowed a grief-storm in your life, and He will give you His strength to rise above it until He ultimately calms it.

When the storms of life come, the wicked are whirled away, but the godly have a lasting foundation.
Proverbs 10:25

---

2. "Are You Struggling?" *Our Daily Bread*, April 7, 2005.

If you feel that soaring above the storm is hard work, uncomfortable, and sometimes downright scary, you are right. That's why I use the analogy of a storm—we might not mind one from a distance, but it's not exactly pleasurable when we're smack-dab in the middle of a big one.

In fact, flying in a storm is extremely dangerous. My cousin Jim knows this from his half-dozen years of soaring into hurricanes and typhoons as part of a U.S. Air Force weather reconnaissance team. It was his team's job to gather weather data so forecasters could better predict a storm's strength.

As a weather reconnaissance team flies together, it's critical that team members trust the "artificial horizon"—a line on the plane's instrument panel that always corresponds to the earth's horizon, no matter which direction the plane is flying.

"When you're in the clouds and in storms and you can't see the horizon—the earth, the ground, good old terra firma—you have to rely on the artificial horizon," Jim explains. "You have to trust that it *is* representing the horizon. You have to trust that it represents something you can't see."

Because of the extreme variability of the weather, there are two government ratings for pilots: one group is cleared to fly only when there's good visibility— following Visual Flight Rules—and the other is cleared to fly even in poor visibility because they can keep a plane controlled solely on the data from their instruments—by Instrument Flight Rules. If you recall after

John F. Kennedy Jr.'s fatal plane crash, the National Transportation Safety Board said the young pilot— who was rated to fly only with Visual Flight Rules— apparently had become disoriented in the night sky and lost control of the plane.[3] Experienced pilots are taught to rely on their instrument panels—no matter how they feel—because they can become so disoriented in clouds or during a storm that they may think they are flying up when they actually are heading down.

In the early days of aviation, when aircraft had few navigational aids, a successful flight was accomplished mainly by the pilot's judgment and instincts; that is, "flying by the seat of their pants."

"Without instruments all you can do is fly by your sensations," Jim explains. "If you are coming out of your seat, you must be upside down. If you are pressed down into your seat, you must be flying higher.

"The problem is that [our perceptions are] not always accurate. You can *feel* like you're flying normal and perfectly fine, but it's just that the airplane is *falling* at just the right speed that feels normal. You have to look at your instruments and believe them."

Flying by the seat of your pants through your grief-storm isn't a good idea either. Feelings can be over-

3. Carl Rochelle, "NTSB: Pilot Disorientation Led to Fatal JFK Jr. Crash," CNN.com, July 6, 2000, http://archives.cnn.com/2000/US/07/06/jfk.crash .report.02/index.html.

powering and paralyzing. You may become so disoriented you don't know whether you're headed up or down.

That's why you need to decide every day to trust the magnetic poles of the earth—in other words, to recognize that God's Word is the compass on your instrument panel in the storm of grief. It is truth, just like the pilot's artificial horizon line, that always will point you in the right direction. And then even better, God's Spirit will give you the strength to move that way.

My friends David and Barry are still trying to comprehend the incomprehensible, but they are not free-falling out of control.

Despite his painful grief, Barry says, "By His strength I keep moving in a positive direction."

David says he finds the greatest relief for his overwhelming feelings of grief when he is reading the Word of God and praying through Scripture.

> *O LORD, do not stay far away! You are my strength; come quickly to my aid!* PSALM 22:19

> *As soon as I pray, you answer me; you encourage me by giving me strength.* PSALM 138:3

> *God is our refuge and strength, always ready to help in times of trouble.* PSALM 46:1

> *I love you, LORD; you are my strength.* PSALM 18:1

You light a lamp for me.
    The LORD, my God, lights up my darkness.
In your strength I can crush an army;
    with my God I can scale any wall. PSALM 18:28-29

God arms me with strength, and he makes my way
perfect. PSALM 18:32

My health may fail, and my spirit may grow weak,
but God remains the strength of my heart; he is mine
forever. PSALM 73:26

I don't know what difficult paths you are facing or
what hard things you must do, but I do know where you
can get the strength to face the unthinkable and even the
seemingly incomprehensible. And I'd like to pray for you
right now from Colossians 1:11-12 in *The Message* para-
phrased version of the Bible:

We pray that you'll have the strength to stick it out over
the long haul—not the grim strength of gritting your
teeth but the glory-strength God gives. It is strength
that endures the unendurable and spills over into joy,
thanking the Father who makes us strong enough to
take part in everything bright and beautiful that he
has for us. Amen.

**TAKE COMFORT: By His strength you can survive your
grief-storm.**

7

SURVIVING THE IMPERFECT STORM

Have you noticed how seemingly insignificant things can bring on a new wave of grief or a fresh batch of tears?

"Every time I look at applesauce, I start to cry," confesses Rita, the member of my grief group with the double heartache of losing her husband and adult son one week apart. "My son, Tommy, loved applesauce, and when I see it, I think of him and cry."

Even a simple trip to Arby's turned into a tearjerker for Rita as she squirted ketchup on her roast beef sandwich just the way she always did for her son when they frequented the fast-food restaurant.

"I just wrapped up my sandwich and left," she says. "I couldn't even stay and eat it because I was so sad."

Rita is not a strange or unusual griever. There's nothing "the matter" with her coping skills. She is experiencing what all grievers seem to notice: grief is much harder than she thought it would be, and certain sights, sounds, smells, and words can trigger intense feelings.

Smelling his aftershave.
Seeing a TV show you used to watch together.
Finding a scrap of paper with her handwriting on it.
Hearing the first notes of her favorite hymn.
Getting out the Christmas lights, which he always
  untangled.

One minute you're coping just fine, and the next minute you're reduced to tears or your legs feel like jelly.

Ralph, a gentleman in my grief group who, like Barry, lost his wife to pancreatic cancer, felt a grief trigger every Friday afternoon. Soon after Carol's death at the age of fifty-seven, he came into my office to chat.

"I'm having a really hard time with all of this," he confessed. "And what's the worst is I can't get out of my mind the time she died. It was about 2:30 p.m. on a Friday, and every Friday at that time I think about her and I just cry and cry."

We reminisced for a long time about his lovely wife, and I could see how real and raw his grief was.

"I can't keep doing this every Friday afternoon—I'm a mess," he told me.

It's times like these I wish I had a Ph.D. in psychology

or at least a manual to fix people's problems. But because I have neither, I simply pray silently and ask the Holy Spirit to give me wisdom far beyond my own limited understanding. And I don't know why, but I continue to be amazed when He does just that.

In an instant I had an idea for Ralph.

"How about trying to remember something else that happened on a Friday afternoon?" I suggested. "If you recall, the Bible says it was about three o'clock on just that day when Jesus died on the cross for you and for me.

"Every Friday a little before three o'clock, why don't you try to remember that is the same time God proved His love for you—and Carol—by allowing His only Son to die so that we can have eternal life? And maybe, just maybe, that time of day could turn into a time of thankfulness."

He loved the idea, and we prayed together that he would have the strength to remember in this new way.

The next time I saw Ralph, he told me Friday afternoons were still hard but much easier now as he thought of Jesus' ultimate sacrifice.

I'm not a psychologist, but I do know that it can help to choose a pleasant memory to associate with a painful one. I did this myself in the early days of dealing with my cancer diagnosis. Every time I looked at the huge scar and twenty-seven staple marks running up my front,

I was faced with an ugly reminder that I had cancer. (And to think I previously had been concerned about a couple of little stretch marks!)

Finally one day as I looked again at my forever-scarred body, I knew I needed a new association for that scar. I decided that I would no longer associate it with *having* cancer but rather with having the surgery necessary to *be healed* from it. My husband and I even went so far as to start celebrating July 2, the day of my cancer surgery, as a new anniversary in our lives—an anniversary of healing. Instead of dreading that emotionally painful reminder of when my world was shaken, I eventually began to look forward to my husband's flower bouquets, encouraging notes, and dinners out. The new association has worked marvelously, and even my daughters have joined in over the years in wishing me a happy "healing anniversary."

When Rita mentioned to our group how sad she was whenever she saw Tommy's favorite applesauce, we suggested that every time she saw it in a store, she buy a case. She could donate it to the local food pantry or even purchase jars of baby applesauce for the crisis pregnancy center.

I pray that you, too, can find some more pleasant associations to attach to your painful memories. If you're having trouble coming up with any, try brainstorming with a trusted friend or a trained counselor. Just don't be surprised when new grief triggers appear months and even years after your loss. Grief is *not* linear—it doesn't start off really strong and then gradually taper off with time. Instead, like a big storm, it can grow larger or smaller in the same day. Psychologists say grievers do best when they go with the ebb and flow of grief and the changing feelings it brings.

"The silliest event does make me cry," admits Mike, the engineer in my group who lost his wife, Annie. "I kept my emotions bottled up before Annie got sick and died. But now I have given myself permission to feel all my feelings, and I do not hold back.

"It's a new experience for me, but I notice I recover a little more quickly when a grief trigger happens," he adds.

I am amazed at my brain's ability to vividly remember some events that happened decades ago yet forget why I just walked into the next room.

For instance, I usually have trouble from one week to the next remembering what I wore to church the week before. It probably doesn't matter (certainly not to God), but I would hate for the congregation to wonder why the senior pastor's wife keeps wearing the same outfit week after week!

On the other hand, I can tell you exactly what I was wearing June 26, 1990, when I went into the hospital for the colonoscopy that revealed my colon cancer. I wore a pale yellow, short-sleeved top with matching yellow slacks and daisy earrings. And after the trauma of that day, I never wore that outfit again, because it reminded me so much of the horrible shock of hearing I had cancer at the age of thirty-six. I didn't bother to get a new association for the outfit; because it was rather old anyway, I simply threw it out!

I'm willing to bet you can vividly recall the events surrounding your loved one's death. What time it was. Where you were. What he or she was wearing. How you reacted.

I've noticed over my years of comforting grievers that everyone's mind seems to be locked in on the details of when his or her world fell apart. (It's a little like how I remember I was off school and playing the Barbie game at my classmate Debbie's house in 1963 when President Kennedy was shot, and how I remember hearing about the first plane hitting the Twin Towers while I was in the chemo room talking with patients.)

I did some reading about why this happens and discovered that researchers think the answer lies in the way our brains process traumatic events.[1] Instead of sending those memories to a part of the brain where most memories are stored, it sort of consolidates them in a different area, where they easily produce vivid flashbacks. Apparently a neurotransmitter that is released during stressful events causes this special "filing" system. Other studies have shown that the brain encodes emotionally charged memories differently than it does mundane

---

1. According to an August 2007 study at McLean Hospital, Boston. The research results were published in *Proceedings of the National Academy of Sciences* 104, no. 35 (August 28, 2007).

ones. That's why we remember our first kiss or scoring the winning touchdown much more easily than what we ate for dinner last Wednesday.[2]

Knowing there's a scientific explanation for these unsettling flashbacks has helped the grievers in my group understand they are not crazy or losing their minds. I hope it does that for you, too.

Still the severity of our mind's and body's responses to grief shocks most grievers. It's not unusual for folks to say that strong emotions, including grief, began even before their loved ones died.

"I went into shock when I heard the diagnosis of cancer," recalls Mike, the widower from my grief group. "I functioned and I took care of Annie, but I was a zombie. I forgot things. The cat lost at least two pounds!"

Terry, a man in my grief group, recalls he "went numb" when the doctor said that Lee, Terry's wife of forty-eight years, wouldn't make it through the night.

Lee actually made it through the night and lived another two months, but Terry's numbness soon gave way to intense feelings of grief as he waited for—and prayed against—the inevitable.

---

2. According to a June 2004 study at Duke University. Florin Dolcos, Kevin S. LaBar, and Roberto Cabeza, "Interaction between the Amygdala and the Medial Temporal Lobe Memory System Predicts Better Memory for Emotional Events," Neuron 42 (June 10, 2004): 855–63.

"I thought God would heal her because we had experienced healing in our family before," Terry explains. "As I was praying for her one day, she said, 'Honey, He's not going to heal me.' I was shocked, but Lee was not—she was so excited that she was going to see Jesus."

Lee's eventual death was no less emotionally painful for Terry even though he already had been grieving for weeks.

"When the time came and she breathed her last breath, I was overwhelmed with emptiness," he says. "I felt God left me; He forsook me. I knew the Word said He would never do that, but it sure felt like He did. . . . I was crushed."

Terry's intense reaction shows just how disorienting a grief-storm can be. Intellectually he knew his feelings were not accurately mirroring God's truth that he knew so well, but he felt them just the same. He was off-course spiritually and having trouble believing his spiritual compass.

Terry got back on track with the help of GriefShare seminars at our church,[3] and then as a regular at our grief group, though he's since moved to Florida to be near his daughter.

"The love, compassion, and oneness of our group was a lifesaver for me," he says. "Our group meetings, devotionals, and prayer times together filled a real void in my life."

Over time as the intensity of his grief lessened, Terry could once again read the Bible and feel God's closeness.

---

3. See GriefShare information in "Grief Care Organizations and Resources" on page 189.

I'm so glad our group could lovingly remind Terry that God's Word is the perfect compass for grievers lost in their storms of sorrow. Now seven years after Lee's death, Terry can honestly say that his relationship "with my wonderful heavenly Father is so much stronger than it was. My walk with Him is much closer and more intimate—He never did leave me or forsake me."

No matter who you are, what you've accomplished, or what you believe, the intensity of your grief probably will surprise you. Perhaps it will help to think of grief as a particular type of storm: the hurricane.

Sebastian Junger, author of *The Perfect Storm*, explains its incredible power: "A mature hurricane is by far the most powerful event on earth; the combined nuclear arsenals of the United States and the former Soviet Union don't contain enough energy to keep a hurricane going for one day. A typical hurricane encompasses a million cubic miles of atmosphere and could provide all the electric power needed by the United States for three or four years. During the Labor Day Hurricane of 1935, winds surpassed 200 miles an hour and people caught outside were sandblasted to death. Rescue workers found nothing but their shoes and belt buckles."[4]

---

4. *The Perfect Storm* (New York: HarperTorch, 1997), 129. One of the most devastating tropical storms in U.S. history, the Labor Day Hurricane hit the Florida Keys and then continued north up the Florida coast.

The death of your loved one is one of—if not *the*—most powerful event you've faced on earth. It's not a "perfect" storm but an imperfect one. And as those in the aftermath of Hurricane Katrina have learned, recovery will take much longer and be more painful than you expect.

"For a time you will be on the emotional 'high seas,' and it's a bumpy ride—one moment intense anger, the next deep sorrow, the next terrifying fear," writes author and educator Daniel Grippo.[5]

The reason you can't "get over" grief or even put it aside for a while is because that would require you to stop loving your loved one. Grief is simply the high price we must pay for love.

This point was driven home to me by a lady in my grief group who called to say she wouldn't be coming to our meetings anymore. I was surprised because I thought she seemed to be fitting in well and enjoying our times together. But she confided that her marriage of more than forty years had not been a very happy one.

"I'm just not really that sad that he's gone," she admitted. "I'm not grieving like the rest of those people are."

She didn't have to pay the high price of love. She already had paid the high price of a miserable marriage.

So when new waves of grief come, I encourage you to remind yourself that your strong grief is a testament to your strong love.

---

5. "Accepting Your Sorrow—Letting Grief Take Its Course," *CareNotes* (St. Meinrad, IN: Abbey Press, 2007).

"When we give sorrow its due," Grippo writes, "sorrow returns the favor by giving us a precious gift—the assurance that we have indeed loved deeply in this lifetime—and that is, without a doubt, one of life's greatest achievements."[6]

> *They wept until they could weep no more.* 1 SAMUEL 30:4

> *My heart is filled with bitter sorrow and unending grief.* ROMANS 9:2

> *Day and night I have only tears for food.* PSALM 42:3

> *Have mercy on me, LORD, for I am in distress. Tears blur my eyes. My body and soul are withering away.* PSALM 31:9

Those verses may describe your grief, or perhaps you even feel as anguished as King David's choir leader, Asaph, did in Psalm 77:

> *When I was in deep trouble,*
>   *I searched for the Lord.*
> *All night long I prayed, with hands lifted toward heaven,*
>   *but my soul was not comforted.*
> *I think of God, and I moan,*
>   *overwhelmed with longing for his help.*

> *You don't let me sleep.*
>   *I am too distressed even to pray!*

---

6. Ibid.

I think of the good old days,
  long since ended,
when my nights were filled with joyful songs.
  I search my soul and ponder the difference now.
Has the Lord rejected me forever?
  Will he never again be kind to me?
Is his unfailing love gone forever?
  Have his promises permanently failed?
Has God forgotten to be gracious?
  Has he slammed the door on his compassion?

PSALM 77:2-9

Notice how Asaph remembers the "good old days" before his world was shaken? But as the psalm continues, Asaph does another kind of remembering:

But then I recall all you have done, O LORD;
  I remember your wonderful deeds of long ago.
They are constantly in my thoughts.
  I cannot stop thinking about your mighty works.

PSALM 77:11-12

Asaph reminds himself of all the blessings he has received from God, and they give him hope that God can once again bring joy—that He has the power to turn the Valley of Weeping into refreshing springs.

I pray that today as you remember and grieve, you also will remember and be grateful. You might want to do what my friend Diana, a young widow now raising her teenage son alone, has done: get a calendar and every evening write down one thing on that date for which you are grateful. That daily dose of thankfulness—although hard to muster some days—has greatly reduced her self-pity, Diana says.

> *And now, dear brothers and sisters, one final thing. Fix your thoughts on what is true, and honorable, and right, and pure, and lovely, and admirable. Think about things that are excellent and worthy of praise. . . .Then the God of peace will be with you.* PHILIPPIANS 4:8-9

TAKE COMFORT: The sorrow you feel in losing your loved one is worth the joy you felt in knowing them.

8

Throwing Rocks at God's Windows

"What did we do to deserve this?"

"When am I ever going to stop reliving those
  last days?"

"Where was God when I prayed for a miracle?"

"Why did she have to die just now?"

"How am I ever going to go on without him?"

"Who really cares how much I'm still hurting?"

I'm sure you could add a million more questions to
these I've heard from grievers. Questions always are wel-
come at our support group, and we often find ourselves
wrestling with God over the injustices we feel. As the
Jewish proverb says: If God lived on earth, people would
break His windows.

Bereavement counselor Robert Zucker explains
the emotional pain so many people feel: "Death may
bring us face to face with a profound sense of injustice,

particularly when we know it to be an untimely or cruel loss."[1]

I'd like to introduce you to a couple of my friends, Gigi and Cindy. They don't know each other, but I've put them together in the same chapter because each has faced an "untimely" and "cruel" loss: Gigi's parents drowned in a freak car accident, and Cindy's sister was abducted and murdered.[2]

Gigi is one of my dearest friends, and I have told her over the years that I would try to include her in every one of the books I write. I put her in my first book as my unnamed friend who often worried about her new "lump of the month." In my second book, I included her by using her last name as a pseudonym for one of our patients. I couldn't quite figure out how to slip her into the inspirational commentary I wrote for the *He Cares* New Testament, but I never dreamed that her world was going to be shaken so much I could write about her "for real" in this book.

On June 13, 2002, Gigi's parents, George and Corla, took a short drive from their Long Island home to a favorite spot on the bay. Every day the elderly couple

---

1. "What I've Learned from Grief," *CareNotes* (St. Meinrad, IN: Abbey Press, 2001).
2. Cindy and her sister Laura's real names have been changed, as have some other details to protect the family's privacy.

took a similar excursion to one of a handful of places where they parked the car so they could "people watch" and enjoy the beautiful waves. They never got out of the car because as George, eighty-eight, often quipped, "I can drive better than I can walk." The next day was their sixty-first wedding anniversary, but only George remembered it. Dementia had robbed Corla of those precious memories long ago, although she still knew and loved her beloved husband and their only child, Gigi. George's face lit up whenever he talked about his wife, still breathtakingly beautiful in his eyes. Corla clung to him in a childlike way—he still was her handsome hero even though his days of rescuing people as part of a city ambulance crew were long gone.

George pulled into the former-dock-turned-parking lot at the only parking spot in the entire lot where there were no wood pilings between the end of the dock and the nearby water. No one knows what happened next, but for some reason George's Jeep Grand Cherokee kept going forward, just fitting between the two dock supports on either side, lurching over the wharf's edge and into the harbor below.

Horrified onlookers watched as the couple beat on the closed car windows and called for help in the sinking car. A bystander rowed out to them, and others tied a rope to a trailer winch and tried to pull the car out of the twelve feet of water. Emergency crews were called, but by the time they reached the couple, George and Corla had been trapped for more than fifteen minutes and had drowned inside the car.

"I never cried so long, so hard, so much in my life," Gigi recalls. "I had to go and look at the car—that was horrible. It still had water in the cup holders."

Her initial reaction included a lot of whys and if onlys.

Why wasn't there a wood piling in front of that parking space? Why did the car just fit between the two dock supports? If only her parents had parked in any other spot. If only help had arrived in time.

It felt incredibly lonely to know she had no immediate family left, Gigi says, but the worst part for her was reliving the awful way her parents drowned, especially because her mother hated to get water in her ears.

"For my parents it was over, but I was still in that car with them," she explains. "I was stuck in those last few moments of their lives."

It was especially hard to ignore the details of the crash as the story was splashed across local newspapers, including the front page of the Long Island edition of *Newsday*. Some misguided friends didn't help either.

"Someone came to my door and told me that 'if God wanted your parents to be rescued, they would have been rescued,'" Gigi recalls. "I thought she had a lot of nerve to say that to me. It's one thing for me to come to that conclusion on my own and another thing for her to prance in and announce it to me."

But Gigi says she finally found peace about the accident as she forced herself to focus on her parents' more than eight decades of living rather than their final fifteen minutes of dying.

"I realized they were so *past* the accident, and I was forgetting everything that had come before," she says.

Cindy has been left with more questions than answers since her older sister Laura's murder just after Easter 2004.

"Our family never really had to ache before this happened; everything was always in place," she explains. "We keep asking: how on earth did this ever happen?"

I never knew Laura because Cindy and I met after Laura's death at a grief seminar I was leading in another state. But through pictures and conversation, I learned she was thirty-five, a marathon runner, an avid whitewater rafter, and a fabulous artist. What I didn't learn— and no one knows—is how she was abducted and why she was murdered.

Cindy and Laura's family celebrated Easter in their parents' northern Virginia home, and then Cindy went to visit her sister for a few days of "girlfriend time."

"We went to a double feature movie, came home and stamped some stationery, and then the next day we visited our favorite quilt shop," Cindy recalls. "She bought some fabric with chili peppers on it and wanted me to make her an apron for her birthday."

But that birthday never came.

Later that morning after Cindy left, someone came to Laura's house, abducted her, shot her four times at close range, and then dumped her body in some nearby woods. One hundred volunteers searched for a week before she was found.

"I totally, totally lost it," Cindy recalls as her tears flow freely once again. "I had so much anxiety, I almost became immobilized."

As the weeks dragged on before an arrest was made in the murder, Cindy's anxiety grew into severe, sleepless depression.[3]

"I kept wondering who killed her and why," she explains.

Depression led to delusion, and Cindy finally was hospitalized for psychiatric treatment. Slowly, through professional counseling, prescription medicines, a prayer vigil at her church, and the support of family and friends, she began to come back to reality.

"You just wonder if you'll ever get back to where you know you need to be," she says.

As we talk almost a year after her sister's death, Cindy happily reports she has found a great deal of emotional healing.

"There's a peace and comfort about me that I don't believe I ever had before," she says. "The ladies in my Bible study really helped when they laid hands on me and prayed for me one night."

She recently finished putting together seven scrapbooks

---

3. Laura's alleged killer is still awaiting trial and facing the death penalty as of this writing.

of Laura's life as gifts for each of her nieces and nephews. Cindy bought a copy of that last movie she and her sister watched together and views it often. She planted 150 daffodils in Laura's memory. She hopes to get a memorial scholarship established at Laura's college alma mater, and, yes, she made the chili pepper fabric apron and wears it in her own kitchen to remember her sister.

Grief is different when a loved one meets a violent end. It raises different kinds of unanswered questions and stirs different emotions than when loved ones die peacefully in their sleep or even when their suffering is mercifully brought to an end by their passing. So where do grievers go with this special kind of pain?

I suggest they run where all those with great suffering need to run: to the only One whose shoulders are broad enough, whose arms are strong enough, and whose love is deep enough.

"It's all right—questions, pain, and stabbing anger can be poured out to the Infinite One and He will not be damaged. . . . For we beat on His chest from within the circle of His arms," writes Susan Lenzkes, author of *When Life Takes What Matters*.[4]

Can you visualize that for yourself? Can you see yourself

---

4. Quoted in Anne Cetas, *Our Daily Bread*, June 25, 2007, http://www.rbc.org/devotionals/our-daily-bread/2007/06/25/devotion.aspx.

crying out your questions to God, beating your clenched fists upon His chest as He holds you in His loving arms?

I am exhausted from crying for help;
    my throat is parched.
My eyes are swollen with weeping,
    waiting for my God to help me. PSALM 69:3

My soul clings to you; your right hand upholds me.
PSALM 63:8, NIV

He tends his flock like a shepherd: He gathers the lambs in his arms and carries them close to his heart. ISAIAH 40:11, NIV

As we cry out to God, some answers may begin to come.

Gigi says she has learned to draw comfort from the fact that "my parents wouldn't have wanted to live without each other.

"We used to worry what we would do if my father died first because with my mother's dementia she would not have understood and she'd experience his death over again a million times a day.

"The only sense I could make of [the accident] is God worked it out and took them both home together," she adds.

Shortly after Laura's murder, her sixty-year-old mother passed away, and in a strange way, it gave Cindy comfort to think of the two of them together with the Lord.

I'm thankful that in spite of life's injustices, neither of my friends wants to throw rocks at God's windows. Instead they have allowed Him to meet them in their grief as they search to make some sense of their loved ones' seemingly senseless deaths.

You've probably already come to realize that no one else can make sense of your suffering for you. People often want to try anyway—they preach about this or that and they tell you why it all happened (like Job's three friends), but they're not God. They can't see the big picture nor do they know the total plan for your loved one's life. I think it makes some people feel better to think they have the answers all figured out. But it certainly doesn't make grievers feel better.

Many of the questions have no acceptable answers anyway. Think about it. Can you think of a single explanation for your loved one's death that would make you say: "That makes so much sense—now I see why there was *no* other way and that they had to die"?

I doubt it. That's why you won't find me trying to give any rationale for your loved one's death. I have plenty of questions for God myself. So come along with me and take your questions to the Almighty. (Bring your rocks if you need to!)

I waited patiently for the LORD to help me, and he turned to me and heard my cry. PSALM 40:1

Listen to my cry for help, my King and my God, for
I pray to no one but you. PSALM 5:2

From the ends of the earth,
    I cry to you for help when my heart is overwhelmed.
Lead me to the towering rock of safety. PSALM 61:2

But after you've hurled your accusations heavenward, don't forget to go to God's Word to find His response. A good place to start might be the promise He gave to Jeremiah, who was filled with so much grief he has been called "the weeping prophet":

I have loved you with an everlasting love;
    I have drawn you with loving-kindness.
I will build you up again
    and you will be rebuilt. JEREMIAH 31:3-4, NIV

I believe God is the only safe person to turn to with your suffering, anger, and pain. He'll give you either the answers you seek or the peace you need to live with the questions. (Besides, broken windows are no big deal to an all-powerful God.)

One of the things I believe God is *unlikely* to do for you is give the rationale for what He did—or didn't do—in your loved one's life. I think it's human nature to wonder why our loved ones had short lives and some other not-so-nice people live long lives. Or why our loved ones met violent deaths while others pass peacefully in their sleep. Or even why the healing we prayed for never came but others got their wishes. I must confess I have a lot of questions for God when I see young mothers in our cancer practice fighting for their lives at the same time elderly folks with dementia in nursing homes are praying to die.

I still don't know the answers to your questions or mine, but something I read in a book by C. S. Lewis has helped me to be more at peace with not knowing.

It's found in a scene from *The Horse and His Boy*, part of Lewis's Chronicles of Narnia. These classic children's books (also loved by adults) are set in the magical land of Narnia, which is ruled by a powerful lion named Aslan (who represents Jesus). At one point Aslan explains to a rich runaway girl named Aravis why some of the awful things that happened to her had to occur. Aravis then asks Aslan what will happen to her stepmother's slave, who was punished for falling asleep after Aravis had drugged her.

"'Will any more harm come to her by what I did?'

"'Child,' said the Lion, 'I am telling you your story, not hers. No-one is told any story but their own.'"[5]

LORD, my heart is not proud;
    my eyes are not haughty.
I don't concern myself with matters too great
    or too awesome for me to grasp.
Instead, I have calmed and quieted myself,

---

5. C. S. Lewis, *The Horse and His Boy* (1954; repr., New York: Harper Collins, 2005), 202.

like a weaned child who no longer cries for its
        mother's milk.
Yes, like a weaned child is my soul within me.
        PSALM 131:1-2

There are so many things I don't understand about the deaths of people I loved. And then I remind myself of the truth of Aslan's words: that no one is told any story but his or her own. (Jesus said something very similar to the disciple Peter after He told Peter some details about his future death but refused to answer Peter's question about how his friend John would die someday.)[6] For the most part I have decided, like the psalmist, not to "concern myself with matters too great or too awesome for me to grasp." But one thing I do understand about the God I love is the undeniable fact that He loves you very much too.

Would you allow me the privilege of praying that you would feel His awesome love for you as you await His healing touch on your broken heart?

> *I pray that from his glorious, unlimited resources he will empower you with inner strength through his Spirit. Then Christ will make his home in your hearts as you trust in him. Your roots will grow down into God's love and keep you strong. And may you have the power to understand, as all God's people should, how wide, how long, how high, and how deep his love is. May you experience the love of Christ, though it is too great to*

---

6. See John 21:18-22

understand fully. Then you will be made complete with all the fullness of life and power that comes from God.

Now all glory to God, who is able, through his mighty power at work within us, to accomplish infinitely more than we might ask or think.[7] Amen.

TAKE COMFORT: You can take all your questions to God because He alone holds the answers.

---

7. Ephesians 3:16-20

9

COMFORTING LIKE NO OTHERS

If you struggle with the fact that God's plan for you included *allowing* deep suffering to touch your life . . . join the club.

When I found out I had cancer, I was pretty upset that God had allowed such a devastating diagnosis to touch me. I desperately wanted to see His miraculous power in my life (i.e., that my colon tumor would disappear before surgery) but was afraid that His plan might be different (i.e., chemotherapy and an uncertain future). I had the distinct sense that my life was about to make a drastic turn, and I wanted to be ahead of the plan and let Him know I wasn't going to go along with it (you know, one step ahead of God!).

I remember lying in my hospital bed before surgery and talking to God, saying: "And don't think You're going to pull me through this somehow and I'm going to go and minister to cancer patients, because I won't do it!"

But a little more than a year later, I started my first Cancer Prayer Support Group. Within five years, I was praying to quit my public relations job and *volunteer* with cancer patients. Less than a year after that, I was employed as a patient advocate in my oncologist's office. Nearly eighteen years later, my life pretty much revolves around ministering to cancer patients. . . . So much for staying one step ahead of God.

What happened to me along the way was that I finally came to terms with the fact that God *had* allowed cancer into my life. He *had* allowed me to suffer with lots of side effects during the chemo. And He *had* allowed me to struggle with discouragement and depression. I finally realized that even though I never would have chosen this path for myself, it *was* my path, and no amount of ranting, raving, weeping, or whining could change it. Either I could keep running from the suffering or I could surrender it to an all-powerful God and believe that somehow, some way, against all odds and my limited logic, He could use it for good.

As I was writing my first book, *When God & Cancer Meet*, I was afraid it might not comfort readers because I struggled with questions about God and didn't have all the answers. The people I wrote about didn't all have fairy-tale endings to their stories either. But you know what? Those things were exactly the reasons readers told me they *did* find solace in the book. God *had* comforted me throughout my awful ordeal, and I could offer others the same comfort He gave me.

So I think that most of us who have suffered—and I am the first to admit that my suffering is *far* less than what my friends in this book and you have probably experienced—are rather reluctant comforters. We would just as soon leave this role to professionals like pastors and counselors or even theologians whom we assume have the answers to hard questions. But I believe God loves to use "wounded healers" to offer comfort to those hurting the most.

I'd like to introduce you to two women who have walked the same unwanted path. Both had to bury a child. The pain and the loss will never go away, but I share their journeys with you so you can see how they have been comforted and how they have allowed God to use them to comfort others.

Matt was the kind of headstrong boy who never wanted to take anybody's word about something. If you told him the sky was blue, Matt needed to go outside just to be sure.

Matt's mother says that "as frustrating as his stubbornness was, it probably was the one thing that kept him alive long after the doctors thought he would die."

She describes her son as a thoughtful and compassionate child who was really good at selecting gifts that pleased others, especially his two brothers.

I distinctly remember the first time I saw Matt. It was

early 1991, and I was sitting in one of the mauve recliners in Dr. Marc Hirsh's chemo room as my weekly IV of toxic chemicals was pouring into my veins. Because I was allergic to the main chemo drug and had to keep taking it anyway (no alternatives existed then), I felt pretty terrible from its side effects. It didn't help that the only antinausea drug available at that time made me terribly sleepy, so I had decided not to take it, in order to function and take care of my three little girls. At thirty-six I was the youngest colon cancer patient Marc had in his year-old practice, and I usually was half the age of everyone else getting treatment. I looked around the chemo room that day, and once again it was "all the old people" and me. I was feeling pretty sorry for myself.

And then five-year-old Matt walked into the room. His head was bald, and I could see some kind of a shunt sticking out of one side of his scalp. His mother was behind him carrying his coat. He climbed up into a recliner, and his little legs swung several inches above the floor.

Hot tears stung my eyes as a small voice in my head whispered: *There's someone younger than you—do you feel better now?*

Lord, forgive me, I quickly prayed. I didn't know the little boy's name, but I began to pray for him, his family, and his uncertain future.

I later learned that Matt had leukemia and was being treated at the National Institutes of Health, about ninety minutes from Marc's office. In order to save traveling time for Matt's family, Marc, under the supervision of NIH, was administering drugs through the brain shunt to try to kill the leukemic cells in Matt's brain and spinal cord.

I had felt sorry for myself because my treatment was scheduled every week for a whole year. Then I heard Matt's treatment lasted *three years*. I was allowed to quit treatment after six months because of my allergic reaction; Matt was never in remission more than eighteen months. He was on chemo during most of his nearly nine-year battle until he passed away just after his fourteenth birthday.

Matt never made it to high school, but his friends kept his memory alive. Throughout their high school years, on every anniversary of his death, Matt's former classmates decorated their lockers with orange and aqua ribbons as a tribute to Matt's love of dolphins—especially the Miami Dolphins pro football team.

To this day, Matt's mom, Elizabeth, describes her grief as "ever changing."

"Sometimes I handle missing Matt fairly well, but even after eight years, I still have days in which I feel like he just died, and I feel the emptiness and sorrow as intensely as if it were just yesterday that he died," she explains.

"One thing that is so difficult to handle is to see everyone else's life go back to 'normal' while I feel like

I'm stuck in a time warp," Elizabeth continues. "While intellectually I understand that Matt's death has less effect on others' lives than on ours and that everyone must move on, I still feel angry and frustrated when I see that happen."

One particular comment that really irritates Elizabeth is the sentiment that everything "will be all right" for her again.

"No, it won't be," she asserts. "A part of my life is missing, and there's nothing all right about that!"

The wound of losing Matt may not bleed as much some days and may even scar over, but it will never be cured and disappear. Elizabeth realizes she is a forever-grieving mother, and I believe that makes her a wonderful wounded healer.

It's why a couple of years ago she was able to comfort the mother of her youngest son Nick's friend, after he was tragically killed in a dirt bike accident.

"I've become a close friend of hers, and we've gone to Compassionate Friends[1] meetings together," Elizabeth says. "She told me that I was a comfort to her because I understood what she was going through even more than her own family did. And I don't act uneasy when she wants to talk about her son, whereas some others try to change the subject. While I don't ever wish someone to lose a child, the fact of the matter is that it happens and God [enables] us to find each other for support," she adds.

---

1. See "Grief Care Organizations and Resources" on page 189.

I doubt that Elizabeth's and my friend Katya's paths will ever cross, as Katya and her family left our area several years ago to move to Israel, but the two women certainly would understand and support each other if they did meet.

Unlike Matt, who lived longer than the doctors predicted, Katya's daughter Zhava (pronounced zuh-HAW-vuh) died just as quickly as medical experts had forecast. And because of the special circumstances surrounding Zhava's life, Katya and her husband's grieving began as soon as she was born.

"When Zhava was alive, we dealt with grief because she was not the healthy child we had expected and because she was not going to be with us very long," Katya explains. "We had to hold her very delicately in our hearts, holding on and letting go at the same time."

Zhava, whose name in Hebrew means "gold," was born with trisomy 18 syndrome[2] and a 90 percent chance she would die within her first year. Trisomy occurs when there is an extra third chromosome in a cell rather than just the normal chromosome pair. (The three most common kinds of trisomy are 18/Edwards syndrome, 13/Patau syndrome, and 21/Down syndrome.) Most children with trisomy 18 have multiple health problems,

2. For more information about this congenital disorder, see http://www.trisomy.org/trisomy18.php.

which make caring for them difficult and physically demanding.

The grief from Zhava's death was *not* what made my friend Katya and her husband, Moshe, compassionate people. They already possessed a special blend of mercy and tenderheartedness, exhibited by the fact that they had unofficially adopted four teenage sisters abandoned by their alcoholic mother after the girls' father died. When Zhava was born in 1988, one of the girls was still living with Katya and her family, which also included four biological children ranging in ages from three to seventeen.

Katya and Moshe gave compassionate care to little hazel-eyed Zhava in hopes of extending her life, but as Katya recalls, "No matter how much loving care I gave her, I watched her life slip through my fingers like water."

"Despite the deep sadness we felt, we welcomed her with open arms," she explains. "We did our best to maintain a normal family life. We took her along with the family to the zoo, on trips, and to congregational activities. We enjoyed every smile she gave us."

Just ten and a half months after her birth, Zhava caught a cold and was hospitalized for about a week. Katya and Moshe were home tending to their other children but felt prompted to go into the hospital at about 10 p.m.

"We got there just in time to be with her before her heart gave out and she died," Katya recalls. "It was a blessing to be there."

Because Katya is such an incredibly compassionate person, almost as soon as Zhava was born, Katya anticipated how her ordeal could be used by God to help others.

"As soon as I realized what I was facing, I prayed the Lord would use this situation to deepen my faith and to touch the lives of others," she says. "I knew that if I had to live through something as painful as this, I wanted to learn as much as I could and not waste any of it."

However, surrendering the situation to God did not mean everything went easily for Katya. After Zhava died, Katya had huge amounts of extra time because she was no longer caring for a special needs child. Her arms and heart ached for the child she could no longer hold and care for.

"For the first time in my life, I found myself dealing with depression," she says. "I was very fragile and often close to tears. I was very sensitive to social situations and to the way I perceived others' reactions to me."

And her grief was complicated by the fact that just before her baby's death in March 1989, Katya became pregnant with twins. Six weeks later she miscarried one twin, but in November she delivered a healthy little girl. Another baby girl was born in 1992, following yet another miscarriage. (Grief experts warn that losses are *not* just mourned separately but often pile up and are dealt with simultaneously.)

"I was dealing with a lot of deaths, one after the other," Katya recalls. "During that time I had to honestly plunge into the grief I was feeling and bring the Lord along with me on these trips.

"Sometimes I was angry at the way people treated me, and I felt as though I had to confront them, which I did," she adds. "However, I also found areas where I had reacted wrongly and treated people unkindly or had expected more from them than they could give. In those cases, I had to ask for forgiveness from them.

"As I moved along this path, I found myself being healed," she says. "I think that this 'grief work' is a major reason why I came through this period of grief as a whole person."

And that is why I believe Katya is a wonderful wounded healer.

"I learned what it was like to have a child die, what it was like to be in emotional pain, and what it was like to be depressed," she explains. "Because of the brief time I had with Zhava and all that I learned from the Lord during this time, I am not afraid to speak about death in a very open way, and I have had many opportunities to reach out to others in dark places.

"In the end my little girl named Zhava truly brought 'gold' into my life and then through me into the lives of others."

Henri Nouwen, the Dutch priest and writer who also taught at Harvard, Yale, and Notre Dame, is the author of a wonderful book entitled *The Wounded Healer*. The book sets out to show how "in our own woundedness, we can become a source of life for others."[3] Nouwen asserts that we don't have to have it all together to minister to others and that our weaknesses (emotional/spiritual wounds) can serve as a source of strength and healing when comforting others.

The Word of God explains it this way:

> *All praise to God, the Father of our Lord Jesus Christ. God is our merciful Father and the source of all comfort. He comforts us in all our troubles so that we can comfort others. When they are troubled, we will be able to give them the same comfort God has given us.*
>
> 2 CORINTHIANS 1:3-4

According to Merriam-Webster's dictionary, the verb *comfort* means "to give strength and hope to" and "to ease the grief or trouble of."[4] That is exactly what God's Word promises the Father God will do for you, so that you, too, can become a comfort to others. He does it by the power of the Holy Spirit, who lives inside all true believers. The Holy Spirit is sometimes even called the Comforter.

> *And I will ask the Father, and another Comforter He will give to you, that he may remain with you—to the age.* JESUS SPEAKING IN JOHN 14:16, YLT

---

3. *The Wounded Healer* (New York: Doubleday, 1979), quote appears on front cover. See page 185 for more details on the book.
4. *Merriam-Webster's Collegiate Dictionary*, 11th ed., s.v. "comfort."

Jesus made those remarks as He talked with His disciples shortly before His death. They already were grieving because He had told them He was going to die very shortly. They couldn't imagine how they would face life without Him. But He assured them that it actually was better that He was leaving because God would send the Holy Spirit, a Comforter, to live inside each of His followers and be with them always. The Spirit's presence would not be limited to a physical body as Jesus was on earth.

> *But I tell you the truth; it is better for you that I go away, for if I may not go away, the Comforter will not come unto you, and if I go on, I will send Him unto you.*
> JESUS SPEAKING IN JOHN 16:7, YLT

That same Holy Spirit Jesus talked about lives inside each follower of Jesus today. He provides the comfort, the help, and the strength that we cannot muster on our own. God promises that a supernatural power from the Holy Spirit will comfort us and then enable us to comfort others. That presence and power are why Proverbs 10:25 can assert that "when the storms of life come, the wicked are whirled away, but the godly have a lasting foundation."

Wouldn't it feel good to sense that supernatural comfort? Wouldn't it feel even better to know your grief has not been wasted—that someone else has felt God's touch through you? Even if you can't imagine how or when that could happen, won't you go to Him today and pray for

His Holy Spirit to soothe, console, calm, and refresh your wounded heart? And then ask Him to bring someone into your life who needs a wounded healer and whom you can comfort by the power of the Holy Spirit, too.

> *Now let your unfailing love comfort me, just as you promised me, your servant.* PSALM 119:76

> LORD, *you know the hopes of the helpless. Surely you will hear their cries and comfort them.* PSALM 10:17

> *I, yes I, am the one who comforts you.* GOD SPEAKING IN ISAIAH 51:12

> *Even though I walk*
>   *through the valley of the shadow of death,*
>   *I will fear no evil,*
>   *for you are with me;*
>   *your rod and your staff,*
>   *they comfort me.* PSALM 23:4, NIV

> *The Sovereign* LORD *has given me his words of wisdom,*
>   *so that I know how to comfort the weary.*
> *Morning by morning he wakens me*
>   *and opens my understanding to his will.* ISAIAH 50:4

I love how *The Message* Bible paraphrases 2 Corinthians 1:3-5, and it is my prayer for you today:

> *All praise to the God and Father of our Master, Jesus the Messiah! Father of all mercy! God of all healing*

counsel! He comes alongside us when we go through hard times, and before you know it, he brings us alongside someone else who is going through hard times so that we can be there for that person just as God was there for us. We have plenty of hard times that come from following the Messiah, but no more so than the good times of his healing comfort—we get a full measure of that, too.

Lord, use us wounded healers to touch someone's life for You. Amen.

TAKE COMFORT: Wounded healers make wonderful comforters, so God will not waste your grief.

10

WONDERING WHAT'S NEXT

Why was my loved one taken from me? You probably still ask this question, even though I doubt you'll get a satisfactory answer in this lifetime.

My friends Brad and Jean Luc were the kind of men I was *sure* God really needed here on earth. Both men sacrificed for years trying to build better lives for some of the world's poorest people. Both men counted it a privilege to serve God and share His love in practical ways. Both men had generous hearts, which inspired them to put others' needs above their own.

But both men died in their forties, leaving behind widows wondering what to do next.

Even though Brad and Jean Luc lived a continent apart and never met, I've put their stories together here because I believe they will give you hope that God can guide you after your loved one's death . . . even when that death doesn't seem to make any sense.

If I had been a passenger on American Airlines Flight 587 on November 12, 2001, it would have calmed my usual plane jitters to know that Pastor Jean Luc also was on that flight. After all, he was considered the leading Haitian pastor in the Dominican Republic and credited with helping start more than twenty new churches and schools for Haitians, the most impoverished people in the Western Hemisphere. He had also recently directed the opening of the area's first hospital to provide quality health care in a Christian context to the Haitian community.[1] I would have felt "safe," certain that God would protect this great man of faith whose labors were touching and changing so many lives. I would have been positive that nothing bad would happen on that flight.

But I would have been very wrong.

Shortly after takeoff from JFK Airport, Flight 587 crashed into a residential neighborhood, killing all 260 people aboard and five others on the ground—making it the second deadliest single-plane accident in U.S. aviation history.[2]

Jean Luc's wife, Elza, says she was at work when the

---

1. The Good Samaritan Mission Council Inc. is a faith-based, ecumenical organization that supports the programs and activities of the Haitian Mission Baptist Church and the Good Samaritan Hospital Foundation. The organization's three major initiatives include construction, medical assistance, and education. Visit http://www.laromana.org to learn more.
2. The deadliest occurred in Chicago in 1979 when 273 people died. September 11, 2001, is of course the deadliest day in U.S. aviation as more than 4,500 people were killed in four separate plane crashes.

news broke. When she arrived home, horrible images from the crash greeted her.

"Usually when I go out, I leave the TV on so people may think there is someone at home, so when I got home, the first thing I saw when I opened the door was a picture of a plane on fire," Elza recalls. "From that moment on, the phone did not stop ringing."

At first the calls were friends wondering if Jean Luc was on the flight, and then the official word came that he was.

"My tears were uncontrollable, and I became inconsolable," Elza says. "I felt as if the world had ended for me. From that moment on, I have felt heartache as if my heart has been bruised, battered, and shattered to pieces. This has been a very sour experience, and I thought I never would recover."

I remember how shocked our church was, too, when we heard the news about Jean Luc. He had visited with us just a few days before while on the East Coast for a meeting with his hospital supporters. Our congregation had been sending volunteer construction crews on annual trips to his hometown of La Romana ever since Hurricane Georges devastated the island in 1998. Now with Jean Luc gone, we wondered how and if the work would continue.

But for Elza there was no question of whether to persist.

"After the death of my husband, many people were asking me if I was going to stay—if I was going to go to the States or back to Haiti," she says. "I told them, 'No, my husband's mission has ended, but not mine.'

"The visions of my husband were my visions as well," she explains. "We worked hand in hand so that we could make our visions a reality."

One of the first projects Elza worked on was their dream of starting a new church on the outskirts of La Romana. Many Haitians had moved from the outlying bateys (villages with shacks serving as homes for the sugarcane company workers) to the closer barrios (suburbs) but still could afford to attend church only occasionally because of the cost of public bus transportation into La Romana, six kilometers away. Elza made "peanut tablets" from roasted peanuts and melted sugar and sold them so she could charter a bus for them to ride free each week until a church could be built in the barrio.

"This area is a place where people have a lot of needs, and I saw that God was placing on my heart the feeling of yearning to stay and work in this area with these people," she explains.

Elza's heart was particularly touched by one mother who moved from the batey to the barrio for a better way of life, but still was so poor she didn't have the basic necessities of life. This mother left her six-year-old son alone for a few minutes so she could search for food at the nearby town dump. Tragedy struck as the little boy was hit and killed attempting to cross the road near his home.

As I write, six years after Jean Luc's death, Elza reports

that construction has started on the Baptist Mission-
ary Church Beraca. (A sister church of ours in York,
Pennsylvania, had the joy of placing the first cement
block!) And in a twist of irony that only God could fore-
see, the new, very simple facility is being constructed at
the former town dump where that young mother scav-
enged for food.

Elza and her team also have started another school
and a medical dispensary. They have purchased a forty-
four-passenger bus to pick up barrio churchgoers as well.
And Elza and her three grown children have initiated
the Jean Luc Phanord Foundation to provide services
such as education, a health center, humanitarian aid, and
a home for the elderly—a rather ambitious task for a
widow wondering what was next.

Elza acknowledges that many times she still wonders
why God allowed Jean Luc to die when so many people
were counting on him.

"Many times I have asked myself that question since
there are so many people who say that if he were here,
things would have gone differently," she says. "However,
I am not one to question God for the things that have
happened, since He is the one who has control of
everything.

"This is how I realized that I should be a strong pillar for those who still needed Jean Luc and counted on
him," she says, adding that she finds great satisfaction
and even joy in continuing her husband's life work.

Elza's faith in God's ability to provide for her and keep

His promises is what has seen her through these lonely years without her life partner.

"God is an almighty God, and He has always opened doors and placed people in my path to help me in this work," she explains. "The Lord has not left me alone but has always been present to help me."

When I look at Elza's life and the obstacles she faces, I am overwhelmed. She describes opposition to their mission work from thieves (the new church's roof has been stolen twice), would-be assassins, and those immersed in witchcraft. She talks of doing construction work by candlelight in some areas that have no running water or electricity.

> *I can do all things through Christ who strengthens me.*
> PHILIPPIANS 4:13, NKJV

That's the verse, the compass on her grief journey, that Elza says keeps her pointed in the right direction.

It's also one that Brad's widow, Connie, considered many times as she wondered how to persevere through her grief.

"I never knew what heartache was until Brad died," Connie says. "I remember praying one day 'just give me five minutes that my heart doesn't ache.'"

While Elza had to board a plane from the Dominican

Republic to the United States to claim her husband's body, Connie had to fly from the United States to Guatemala for the same grim task.

Brad and Connie, both in their late forties, had never been able to have children but believed their circumstances gave them the opportunity to "adopt" some of the world's poorest children as their own. They used all their vacation time to volunteer at children's hospitals and orphanages in Russia, Belize, Honduras, and Guatemala. Brad, an easygoing guy with a boyish grin, was on his annual two-week visit to a Guatemalan orphanage doing light construction work when he collapsed without warning. He literally was working beside and chatting with a fellow volunteer one minute and then gone the next. Despite the resuscitation attempts of nearby nurses, he could not be revived. The Guatemalan death certificate listed heart attack as the cause of death.

Within hours of receiving word of Brad's death, Connie started journaling, or as she calls it, "putting my prayers to paper." Over the ensuing months and years, she filled more than nine hundred notebook pages with details of her heart-wrenching journey, and she graciously allowed me to view these grief glimpses, including her very first entry:

> 9-28-04, 5:15 a.m. Oh Jesus—This is the most painful place I have ever been—for the past 14 hours I feel like I have been forced to live out a part in a play that I do not want to be in. And yet I do not get to

choose. For whatever reason, for whatever purpose, you chose Monday, 9-27-04 as the day to call Brad home to be with you forever. And yet on the same day, my whole world is turned upside down—no, that's too clean cut. My whole world is destroyed. My best friend, my soul mate and life partner has been permanently removed from my life. There is an unending ache in my heart and I just keep saying over and over again, "I just want him to come home—I just want to see him again."

About two weeks later, Connie says she "happened upon" Psalm 62 in her daily Bible reading.

> *Find rest, O my soul, in God alone;*
> *my hope comes from him. . . .*
> *Trust in him at all times, O people;*
> *pour out your hearts to him,*
> *for God is our refuge.* PSALM 62:5, 8, NIV

"I read that psalm every day for over a year," she says. "I knew that my hope didn't come from Brad or my family or friends; it came from God—no one else, nowhere else, nothing else.

"I needed to stay fully focused on God and instruct my soul to do so too," she explains. "I knew I had to go to God's Word for answers."

And that is how God began to meet Connie in her grief. She kept going to His Word for answers and then jotting down the things He was teaching her. Very simply she believed God could supply what she needed to survive each moment. As Connie read the Scriptures, she began applying them in prayer to her own life.

> The LORD your God is with you,
>   he is mighty to save.
>   He will take great delight in you,
>   he will quiet you with his love. ZEPHANIAH 3:17, NIV

Lord, I need you to quiet me with your love—I'm unraveling, she prayed.

> Though he brings grief, he also shows compassion
>   because of the greatness of his unfailing love.
> For he does not enjoy hurting people
>   or causing them sorrow. LAMENTATIONS 3:32-33

Lord, I have the same overwhelmingly anxious feeling that I've had every single day since Brad died, she prayed. *Jesus, meet me in the pain today.*

The emotional pain was amplified by the frustrations Connie felt in trying to take care of everything at their home, especially the yard work. She and Brad already had downsized to a smaller home when they cut back his work schedule so he could do more volunteer missions, but their tiny backyard was basically a mass of unmanageable ivy. So she asked a landscaper from her church (who had done a really nice job on some work in the front yard the summer before) if he had any suggestions.

The landscaper suggested building a "pocket of peace" in the backyard, which would give Connie time and space for God to meet her grief. She liked the idea and was especially thrilled when the landscaper told her he wanted to design it "in a way that would honor the Lord, honor you, and honor Brad."

The landscaper was true to his word and built a beautiful little patio with a wall behind it and small terraced gardens above it. If you looked carefully, you could see small stone crosses standing in the gardens that had been custom made to match the wall—a reminder to Connie to look to the Lord because her help would come from Him. It was a perfect pocket of peace.

> *I lift up my eyes to the hills—*
> *where does my help come from?*
> *My help comes from the LORD,*
> *the Maker of heaven and earth.* PSALM 121:1-2, NIV

Connie sat there each day reading her Bible and pouring out her heart to her heavenly Father. As she did, she says she began to understand the difference between being *resigned* to Brad's death and being *surrendered* to it and whatever was next.

"If you're resigned, you don't have a choice," she explains. "But if you're surrendered, you choose to yield yourself.

"I started really surrendering myself to God," she says.

"I told God, 'I will yield to your plan—I don't have to understand it. You are either sovereign or You're not—You can't be partially sovereign.'"

And as God's peace poured into her heart, Connie was about to find out that God had another plan for her life—one she had never imagined or even thought she wanted.

Did I mention that the landscaper was tall, dark, handsome, and single?

Despite the fact that Connie was resolute on never marrying again or even "needing" someone in her life, some of Connie's closest friends and even her mother were praying that God might bless her with another love. In retrospect, Connie says she thinks her isolation mind-set was an act of self-protection because she did not want to "get hurt like that again."

"Getting married again was not even on the radar," Connie recalls. "I felt I had my gift [in Brad] and I would go the rest of the way by myself."

But slowly what began as a business relationship turned into a friendship and then blossomed into full-blown love.

"I couldn't imagine why on earth God would give me another love like that," Connie says, "but a friend said to me, 'God loves you—what makes you think He wouldn't do it a million times?'"

So three years after Brad's death, Greg, the landscaper, became Greg, Connie's husband. And as one more reminder of His love for her, God blessed Connie with a son, fifteen, and a daughter, twelve, whom Greg had been raising alone for the previous decade. The kids heartily agreed with their dad's decision to remarry. His daughter, Victoria, was even there for the marriage proposal when Connie "found" her engagement ring in a tackle box during a family fishing expedition.

Victoria actually helped plan the whole proposal, and her excitement showed as she told Connie: "When 'we' get married, you won't have to go home anymore, and we'll be a family." (I love how she used the word *we*! She obviously felt such a part of the whole marriage.)

I know Connie will never forget the painful loss of Brad, but I also know she has seen Romans 8:28 in action:

> *And we know that God causes everything to work together for the good of those who love God and are called according to his purpose for them.*

Both Connie and Elza have had front-row seats watching God turn their Valleys of Weeping into places of refreshing springs. Does it mean they'll never shed another tear for their departed husbands? Hardly. Does it mean they'll stop wondering how and why God's plan had to work out the way it did? I doubt it. Does it mean that in spite of their great grief, they have found God has good intentions for their lives? You better believe it.

> *To all who mourn in Israel,*
> *he will give a crown of beauty for ashes,*
> *a joyous blessing instead of mourning,*
> *festive praise instead of despair.* ISAIAH 61:3

No matter how much you have lost or how little you have left, God can make something good come from it. The Bible says He is the God "who creates new things out of nothing" (Romans 4:17).

When God promised Abraham he would become "the father of many nations," Abraham had no children and both he and his wife were too old to start a family. The promise did not make sense. But "even when there was no reason for hope, Abraham kept hoping" (Romans 4:18).

Can you dare to hope today? Even if there's no earthly reason, no logic from a human perspective, can you dare to hope that God can create new things out of nothing? Will you surrender—not resign—yourself to His plan and trust He will show you what's next?

That's what He's done for both Elza and Connie— giving one the courage to continue on a difficult path, the other the peace to forge a new one, and both a grateful joy that permeates their sorrow.

> *You have turned my mourning into joyful dancing.*
> *You have taken away my clothes of mourning and*
> *clothed me with joy,*
> *that I might sing praises to you and not be silent.*
> *O LORD my God, I will give you thanks forever!*
> PSALM 30:11-12

TAKE COMFORT: God can create beauty from ashes, turn mourning into dancing, and change weeping into joy.

11

Hoping for Heaven

In my office, I have a file drawer full of my notes on the hundreds of patients I've met in our cancer practice who have passed away. When I have to look in that drawer, waves of grief often sweep over me as I see the names of those I have loved and lost. I am especially saddened by the young mothers who didn't get to see their children grow up—probably because that was my greatest fear when I, too, faced that dreaded disease.

One of the hardest of those young mothers to lose was my dear friend Melina. Even now as I look at her beautiful smiling face on the cover of her memorial service bulletin, I cannot stop the rush of hot, stinging tears.

I'd like to share a little of Melina's life with you, but mostly I'd like to share Melina's Hope with you. Her life—and her death—both have a message for those I call the "believing-grieving."

Melina was a dark-haired, dark-eyed beauty (think full-blooded Italian parents). She and her husband, Brian, met in 1988 and married a decade later. Together their love produced two adorable little girls, Cecilia and Olivia. Melina was a mortgage broker, and Brian worked as an electrical engineer.

It was a beautiful world.

But that was before October 2003 came and with it a diagnosis of Stage III colon cancer for thirty-three-year-old Melina. I had just met Melina's younger sister Rina through a mutual friend, and I sent Melina a little note of encouragement when I heard about her diagnosis. I knew how important it is to hear from other survivors of "your" kind of cancer. I reminded her that I was still alive after having colon cancer spread to *five* lymph nodes (she had it in "only" two).

After surgery, Melina started chemotherapy, availing herself of the new anti–colon cancer drugs that had not been available to me back in 1990. But in August 2004, three weeks after doctors told her there was no evidence of disease, she developed terrible abdominal pain: tests revealed a grapefruit-sized mass on her ovary. Then a PET scan showed tiny cancerous spots in both lungs.

Melina quit her job to stay home with her daughters, and for nearly three more years, she fought back against the cancer, enduring such things as a clinical trial that left her bedridden for five months and a trip to Germany for a new laser procedure to remove the lung nodules. She spent two weeks in California learning about organic and whole food nutrition, and traveled to cancer centers in Philadelphia and Virginia to see what they could offer.

Each new approach seemed to knock down the cancer for a while, only for it to rear its ugly head once again.

Like many cancer patients, Melina started a Web site. She called it Melina's Hope.[1] As an author who appreciates a really great opening thought, I loved the way Melina began the first page of her site: "You might think my hope is to preserve my earthly life. . . ."

That's exactly what I was thinking her hope would be. But that's because I was thinking of her cancer diagnosis as the beginning of her story. She set me and all her readers straight right away: "My story begins one Sunday morning in August 2002.

"What a beautiful day," she writes. "It was the day I accepted the Lord Jesus into my heart. With that acceptance came a promise: if I trust the Lord with all my heart and acknowledge Him in all my ways, He would direct my paths—and that He did in my journey with colon cancer."

And that is why Melina said her strongest hope was not to preserve her earthly life, "but more important than that, is my hope that my story changes but one heart to

---

1. See http://www.melinashope.com.

accept the love and protection that comes from our Lord Jesus Christ."

> *Trust in the LORD with all your heart;*
> *do not depend on your own understanding.*
> *Seek his will in all you do,*
> *and he will show you which path to take.*
>
> PROVERBS 3:5-6

That was Melina's favorite verse—the one on which she firmly staked her life and the one by which she squarely faced her death.

"I can't, however, abandon the one true healer, our Lord Jesus Christ," she wrote on her Web site about five months before her passing. "It's His decision where my healing will take place, here on earth or with Him in heaven. That is where my hope and comfort come from. I trust completely that the Lord will do what is best for me, my family and friends."

Even though Melina grieved because she was going to leave this earth and not see her little girls grow up, or grow old with her husband, she had hope because she knew this life is not all there is.

> Hope that she was not saying good-bye forever.
> Hope that she was headed to her real home:
> Heaven.
> Hope that in Heaven she would get a new, disease-
> free body.

Hope that one day there would be a grand reunion
of all her family and friends who also trusted in
the Lord.

Hope that grieving for the believing is not the same
as it is for those who have no hope.

The Bible makes it very clear that believers in Jesus have
an eternal hope that transcends all our present sorrow
and changes the way we view the future.

> *And now, dear brothers and sisters, we want you to know*
> *what will happen to the believers who have died so you*
> *will not grieve like people who have no hope. For since we*
> *believe that Jesus died and was raised to life again, we*
> *also believe that when Jesus returns, God will bring back*
> *with him the believers who have died. . . . So encourage*
> *each other with these words.* 1 THESSALONIANS 4:13-14, 18

The Bible says grieving is different for the believing;
we don't grieve "like people who have no hope." While
it's terribly hard to be the people left behind, we have
the firm assurance that our believing loved ones have
been healed in Heaven and we will be together with
them again one day.

> *Jesus told her, "I am the resurrection and the life.*
> *Anyone who believes in me will live, even after dying.*

Everyone who lives in me and believes in me will never ever die." JOHN 11:25-26

Melina's husband, Brian, says he experiences this difference as he struggles to raise their daughters, five and seven, without his wife by his side.

"As sad as I am that I am without my best friend, I am so happy that she is in Heaven," he says. "You experience excruciating heartache from the finality of death, and no matter what you do, you cannot get away from it. But at the same time, you know without one shred of doubt that they are in Heaven—I can't help but be happy for Melina.

"I think God gives clarity to believers who suffer loss," Brian continues. "The clarity for me is that Melina's dying is not the thing to dwell on, but that she is alive in Heaven."

I love how Brian always capitalizes *Heaven*—I do, too, because it's a *real* place, as real as Chicago or California or Cancun. I used to have an inaccurate view of Heaven as a place with nothing but fluffy white clouds, streets of gold, harp strumming, and twenty-four-hour singing. I love to praise God (at least with a "joyful noise") but *never-ending* singing, I must admit, sounded rather boring. I'm so glad I read Randy Alcorn's book *Heaven* and got a true, biblical view of my future home.

"[I]n order to get a picture of Heaven—which will one day be centered on the New Earth—you don't need to look up at the clouds; you simply need to look around you and imagine what all this would be like without sin and death and suffering and corruption," writes Alcorn, who has thoroughly studied what the Bible says about Heaven. "I imagine our first glimpse of Heaven will cause us to . . . gasp in amazement and delight. That first gasp will likely be followed by many more as we continually encounter new sights in that endlessly wonderful place."[2]

Alcorn goes on to describe Heaven as full of gardens, cities, and kingdoms, where we will continually praise God *while* we fellowship with others, create, learn, and perhaps even invent! Since I read his marvelous book, I have had a longing for Heaven as never before.

Alcorn continues:

> Think of friends or family who loved Jesus and are with him now. Picture them with you, walking together in this place. All of you have powerful bodies, stronger than those of an Olympic decathlete. You are laughing, playing, talking, and reminiscing. You reach up to a tree to pick an apple or orange. You take a bite. It's so sweet that it's startling. You've never tasted anything so good. Now you see someone coming toward you. It's Jesus, with a big smile on his face. You fall to your knees in worship. He pulls you up and embraces you.

2. Randy Alcorn, *Heaven* (Carol Stream, IL: Tyndale House Publishers, 2004), 17.

At last you are with the person you were made for, in the place you were made to be.[3]

I wept tears of joy the first time I read that passage. What an awesome reunion that will be.

But what if you don't have the assurance that your loved one was a believer in Jesus?

I would be deceiving you if I didn't say that the Bible clearly states that eternal life—Heaven—is promised only for those who have a relationship with God through His Son, Jesus, the Messiah.

> *Jesus told him, "I am the way, the truth, and the life. No one can come to the Father except through me."*
> JOHN 14:6

> *"There is salvation in no one else! God has given no other name under heaven by which we must be saved."*
> THE APOSTLE PETER SPEAKING ABOUT JESUS IN ACTS 4:12

My friends Joyce and Tod, whom you'll learn more about in chapter 13, admit they are not 100 percent sure about their deceased son Tim's eternal destiny.

"I feel Tim knew the Lord as a young child, but

---

3. Ibid., 18.

whether he's in Heaven, I don't know for sure," Joyce says. "He wrote on his [suicide] note, 'I'll see you in Heaven.' He knew he couldn't say that unless he was right with God."

Joyce says she copes with her uncertainty by focusing *not* on what she doesn't know about her son, but on what she does know about her heavenly Father.

> God loves each and every one of us. (John 3:16)
> God doesn't want a single person to perish.
>   (2 Peter 3:9)
> God knows the heart of every person. (Psalm 44:21;
>   1 John 3:19-20)
> God can save anyone. (Luke 1:37)
> God will save anyone who calls on His name.
>   (Romans 10:13)

Do you think the family of the thief on the cross next to Jesus knew he had put his faith in the Son of God at the very last minute? He called out to Jesus with one of his last breaths, and Jesus assured that repentant, convicted felon that "today you will be with me in paradise."[4] Perhaps his family grieved as if there was no hope for him. Imagine the surprise of the thief's believing relatives when they got to Heaven and he was there to greet them!

If you are unsure about your loved one's faith, I pray you can entrust your doubt—and his or her soul—to the One who loves him or her most. And I also pray that you

---

4. Luke 23:39-43

won't have any such doubts about your own relationship with Jesus and your eternal destiny.

Brian has none.

"The night Melina left this earth, Heaven's population grew by one," Brian says. "Through all my pain and sorrow from losing Melina, I know that God wants us in Heaven and that I will join her there one day."

Eternal life is a gift—free to us by faith—but very costly to Jesus, who paid for our sins by dying on the cross.[5] It's the gift that Melina received in August 2002, which made her one of the believing-grieving. It enabled her—and her husband—to face her death from an eternal, not earthly, perspective. It's the gift—the hope—she prayed others would find too. Hear again the hope of a dying young woman: "My hope [is] that my story changes but one heart to accept the love and protection that comes from our Lord Jesus Christ."

Perhaps it was a hope for you.

I am so grateful that Melina and I are "forever friends" even though we have to be separated for a little while. Near the very end of her life, she told her distraught adult family members: "I know you guys don't want to hear this, but I know where I'm going and I can't wait to get there!"

5. Ephesians 2:8-9

Then she added with a smile: "You'll see me again."

One of my favorite daydreams is to imagine that upon my arrival in Heaven, Jesus greets me and then takes me to a long line of smiling people: Melina and all of the faith-filled cancer patients I knew. I see that they are physically healed just like we prayed for so many times. We embrace, and while there are no *sad* tears in Heaven, in my daydream, I overflow with tears of joy.

But my dream is not just wishful thinking. The promise of Heaven for all who believe in Jesus is real, and I know that reunion will really happen.

One of the people I look forward to meeting in Heaven is someone I never knew on earth: my paternal great-grandmother, Mary Andrews Peirce. She was a prolific poet, and I'd like to think my writing ability came through her genes. In 1928 when she was nearly sixty, she wrote a poem she called "HOME."

> *In childhood's days, our thoughts of Heaven*
> *Are pearly gates, and streets of gold.*
> *But in the gathering years,*
> *When time, within its fading leaf*
> *With eyes, perchance be-dimmed with tears,*
> *And hearts oft' overwhelmed with grief,*
> *We look beyond the pearly gates,*
> *Beyond the clouds of sin's dark night,*
> *And see a place where loved ones wait,*
> *A place all beautiful and bright.*
> *And over all, we'll see the face of Him*

Who'll bring us to our own—
Not to some far-off, distant place.
For Heaven is, after all, just HOME.

My prayer for you today is Romans 15:13:

I pray that God, the source of hope, will fill you
completely with joy and peace because you trust in him.
Then you will overflow with confident hope through the
power of the Holy Spirit. Amen.

TAKE COMFORT: The believing-grieving have a sure hope that forever changes everything.

12

Going On before Us

Is any particular part of the day most difficult for you? Some grievers tell me they dread too-quiet evenings at home. Some say looking at an empty chair at mealtimes is especially hard. Still others hate bedtime. Many say that morning is the worst, as each sunrise brings another day of mourning. Special occasions like holidays can add another layer of sadness for those left behind.

My friend Connie wrote this poignant entry in her journal, just three months after her husband's death: "12:40 a.m. 12/25/04—It's Christmas. It's really here and Brad really isn't here. Not just for today, but for any Christmas again and that makes me so sad."

Connie and the grievers I know all say they were woefully unprepared for just how much they would miss their loved ones. Some say they feel a new wave of sorrow at every "first" special occasion after their loved ones' passing—first birthday, first Thanksgiving, first wedding anniversary, first vacation, first anniversary of their death.

But other mourners say these special days are not really any more arduous than all the other mundane dates—every day is painful. Nearly all of the grievers in my support group are widows and widowers who were married forty or fifty—some even sixty—years. And each new day not only exacts an emotional toll but also gives rise to many practical problems.

"I didn't know how to iron, and I didn't think I could do it," says Jim, a retired engineer married nearly sixty years. "I finally figured it out, but I know for sure I hate 100 percent cotton!" he adds as he shakes his head in disgust over his wrinkle-challenged shirts.

Just putting a meal on the table is admittedly quite an ordeal for most of the men in my group. Mike, another widowed engineer who had been married to a great cook, says he tried to make lasagna with Swiss and American cheeses.

"I found out that doesn't work—you have to go out and buy ricotta cheese," he says with a laugh.

In addition to ironing, Jim says he's working on mastering his wife's Crock-Pot and her bread machine. "I'm not much of a chef," he says. "It's more like survival cooking."

"You'll get better," offers his friend Charlie B., whose wife has been gone much longer than Jim's. (I believe him because I've tasted Charlie's homemade soup and angel food cake!)

Many people assume that the first year of grief is the hardest, but that is not always true. If you are past that first-year mark and things are getting easier, be grateful. But if life seems even harder, you are not alone. Sometimes those first twelve months don't seem to be all that bad and then—*pow!*—the sorrow really hits.

"The second year was the worst for me," says my friend Linda, widowed now for four years. "I think the first year I was just in shock and didn't feel it as much."

And while some of the intense emotions surfaced later, the financial concerns hit almost immediately. Linda's husband, Mike, had been the major bread-winner, and she was left without his income or a pension. Then shortly after his death, she lost her part-time job as a hairdresser.

"I worried whether I would be able to afford to live on my own," she says. "I'm only sixty-three years old—I can't be drawing out all the money we saved. What will I do when I'm seventy or eighty?"

Thankfully Linda's brother is an accountant and helped her navigate the financial world. She also found another hairdresser job, which she loves. The money worries she feared after Mike's death have not material-ized, and she is managing on her own. She even has a little cash left that she can use to dote on the two pre-cious grandsons born since Mike's passing!

Facing each new day—although still difficult—defi-nitely has gotten easier. "I always wonder, *How am I ever going to pay all these bills?* but it works out somehow," she says. "I always have enough, and my new job has worked out even better than my old one. I know God is definitely watching out for me!"

> *No eye has seen, no ear has heard,*
> *and no mind has imagined*
> *what God has prepared*
> *for those who love him.* 1 CORINTHIANS 2:9

I hope that's a verse you'll remember as you face another day without your loved one. Repeat it when you climb out of bed in the morning or when you crawl back in at night. Recall it at mealtimes or holidays or anytime the dread rises in your aching heart.

You are *not* just stumbling through life without purpose or peace. You may feel unprepared, but God *is* prepared and He is preparing things for you—good things—things that you can't even imagine. I believe He literally goes before all of His followers into each new day to provide what we'll need for that day. Hear His promise through Moses' words in Deuteronomy 31:8 (as expressed in three different Bible versions):

> *The LORD himself goes before you and will be with you;*
> *he will never leave you nor forsake you. Do not be afraid;*
> *do not be discouraged.* NIV

*GOD is striding ahead of you. He's right there with you.
He won't let you down; he won't leave you. Don't be
intimidated. Don't worry.* THE MESSAGE

*Do not be afraid or discouraged, for the LORD will
personally go ahead of you. He will be with you; he
will neither fail you nor abandon you.* NLT

Authors Henry and Richard Blackaby explain God's
promise this way:

> God never sends you into a situation alone. He
> always goes before His children, as He did with the
> children of Israel when He led them with a cloud
> by day and a pillar of fire by night. . . . He always
> precedes you in any situation you encounter. God is
> never caught by surprise by your experience; He has
> already been there. He is prepared to meet every
> need because He has gone before you and knows
> exactly what you will need for your pilgrimage.[1]

And the really good news is that He doesn't just go
on ahead of us, He stays *with* us, too, ensuring we are
never alone.

"Not only does God go *before* you, but He also stands
beside you and *behind* you, to provide protection and

---

1. Henry T. Blackaby and Richard Blackaby, *Experiencing God Day by
Day: Devotional* (Nashville: B & H Publishing, 1998), 94. The story of
the Israelites being led by God with a cloud and a fire pillar is found in
Exodus 13:21.

comfort," the Blackabys add. "If you are going through a difficult or confusing time, know that your Lord has gone before you and He is present with you. He is fully aware of what you are facing, and He is actively respond-ing to your need."[2]

God knows Jim needs to learn how to iron (and hates 100 percent cotton!). He knows Mike needs to discover new cheeses. He knows just how much money Linda needs. And God knows exactly what you need to be prepared for today.

He knows and He has gone before you to provide it. All He asks of you is to have faith.

Have faith.

Just trust.

Such simple phrases, but ones that are so difficult to put into practice at times.

It's often hard for me to "have faith" and "just trust" because I'm a task-oriented, logical person who wants to rationalize and work things out myself. I remember once even trying to talk my middle daughter, Bethany, *out* of having so much faith.

She was four and getting ready to attend her second year of preschool. It was only a three-month preschool class, which met for a couple of hours twice a week as part of a child education class at our local high school. (The sole cost was twenty-five cents, for the daily snack!) Bethany had enjoyed the class the year before because

2. Ibid.

of the special friendship she'd made with her student-helper, Missy.

"I'm going to pray that Missy will be my helper this year," she announced at bedtime a couple of weeks before preschool started.

I gently explained to her that Missy could not be her helper because she was in the class *last* year and students rarely took a second year of the class. And even if Missy did, the teacher had told me she always made sure *not* to give the preschoolers the same helper.

"I'm praying that Missy will be my helper," Bethany insisted, completely undeterred by my logical explanation.

This dialogue continued night after night: Bethany would pray for Missy to be her helper, and then I'd explain why that wasn't going to happen. The whole scenario had me concerned because, at the time, Bethany was very shy (though she eventually overcame that and was voted "Most Comical" in her high school graduating class). She had been extremely reticent about the preschool experience the previous year until Missy came to her rescue. I knew this year could be tougher for Bethany because her big sister Danielle was now a kindergartner and wouldn't be in preschool with her. I kept praying that God would provide another good helper for Bethany and that she would enjoy herself again.

Imagine my surprise when I picked up Bethany after the first day of preschool and she ran toward the door holding hands with Missy.

"I told you Missy would be my special helper!" she announced with a huge grin on her little freckled face.

The preschool teacher appeared very flustered, apologizing profusely to me for her "mistake" in giving Bethany the same helper.

"I don't know how this happened—I always make sure not to do that," she said. "I'll change it right away."

"Don't even think about it," I quickly replied. "You were the answer to my child's prayers."

> *You go before me and follow me. You place your hand of blessing on my head.* PSALM 139:5

Do I believe God will always answer our prayers exactly the way we hope? You have to be kidding. Do I believe that if we have "enough" faith, we'll get exactly what we want? I think you know me well enough by now to know that can't be true. So what *does* it mean to have faith that God will provide?

I think author Jennifer Kennedy Dean explains what faith is—and isn't—as well as anyone I've read:

> Faith is not believing real hard. Faith is not shutting your eyes and drawing a long breath and willing yourself to believe something. You can make yourself believe anything, true or not. Believing it won't make God do it. Belief is one thing; faith is something else.

Because many believers have mistaken belief for faith, they have had experiences in prayer that are discouraging and disappointing. They have believed with all their might that God would perform in a certain way that seemed best to the pray-er. . . .

Friends, it won't work. No matter what you do, you will never be able to manipulate God. . . . Faith is not knowing *how* God will bring His will into being; faith is knowing *that* God will bring His will into being.[3]

Do you have that kind of faith today? Do you have faith that God will be faithful even though life has been unfair and your loved one has died? Do you have faith that He personally has gone before you into this day and will provide what you need for each moment? Do you have faith that when God meets your grief, He can guide you like no other? You may be disappointed when you put your faith in a specific outcome, but you *never* will be disappointed when you put your faith in the Lord.[4] Have faith in Him.

If your present seems precarious or your future feels frightening, your compass, God's Word, has a message just for you:

3. *Live a Praying Life* (Sarasota, FL: The Master's Touch Publishing Company, 1998), 120 (italics in original).
4. "For the Scripture says, 'Whoever believes in him will not be disappointed'" (Romans 10:11, NASB).

The LORD says, "I will guide you along the best pathway
 for your life.
 I will advise you and watch over you." PSALM 32:8

The LORD will guide you continually,
 giving you water when you are dry
 and restoring your strength.
You will be like a well-watered garden,
 like an ever-flowing spring. ISAIAH 58:11

Because of God's tender mercy,
 the morning light from heaven is about to break
  upon us,
to give light to those who sit in darkness and in the
 shadow of death,
  and to guide us to the path of peace. LUKE 1:78-79

For that is what God is like. He is our God forever and
ever, and he will guide us until we die. PSALM 48:14

You might have been unprepared for your loved
one's death, and you may feel ill-prepared for your
life without him or her, but the consistent message of
Scripture is that God is prepared and preparing as He
goes before us.

Think about some of Jesus' last words to His fearful
disciples shortly before His death:

Don't let your hearts be troubled. Trust in God, and
trust also in me. There is more than enough room in

my Father's home. If this were not so, would I have told
you that I am going to prepare a place for you? When
everything is ready, I will come and get you, so that you
will always be with me where I am. John 14:1-3

Jesus has gone before us to prepare a place for all
true believers in Him and is coming back to take us
there someday.

So what does it mean for grievers as God goes before us
into each day? I think it means He lights our way, guiding
us in our decision making; and He makes a way, giving us
strength to do what we didn't think we could. Sometimes
He miraculously clears a path for us (as He did for my
Bethany). Sometimes He gives us the strength to clear
our own paths (like Jim learning to cook), and sometimes
He brings others alongside us to make a way (like Linda's
brother helping her with finances).

And sometimes He creates "coincidences" to convince
us that He really has gone before us. My friend Barry,
whom you met several chapters ago, talks about an experience he had shortly after his wife Barb's death. It wonder-
fully illustrates God's orchestrating power.

Barry and his family were at the beach in Ocean City,
New Jersey, on Barb's July 16 birthday—the first one
since her passing in February. What normally would
have been a joyous celebration was now a day they all
dreaded as one more glaring reminder that she was no

longer with them. Even though they were on vacation, Barry decided to go to worship, so they drove to a fairly large church nearby.

"A lady at the door gave me a big smile when we came in and said I looked like I needed a 'special hug,'" recalls Barry.

Barry and his family then took their seats. As he looked at the front of the worship bulletin, he saw a quote from Psalm 139—the same chapter Barry had read to his family as his wife lay dying.

"I said, 'Wow, that's pretty neat!' and then I opened the bulletin and saw we were going to sing 'Knowing You.'"[5] That was the song the family had tearfully sung at Barb's memorial service.

And then the crowning "coincidence" came when the pastor began the service and reminded everyone it was a parishioner's birthday—the lady at the door who had hugged Barry as he came in.

"I was thinking, *Whoa, hold it, this is too much*," recalls Barry. "The verses, the song, and then the same birthday as Barb's—it was amazing!"

His beloved Barb is still gone and still missed, but Barry doesn't doubt for a moment that God went before him on that difficult day and provided a reminder of His love and care for Barb's family.

---

5. Graham Kendrick, "Knowing You," 1993, Make Way Music, www.grahamkendrick.co.uk. If you're not familiar with this beautiful chorus, part of the lyrics read, "Knowing You, Jesus / Knowing You, there is no greater thing."

But when God goes before you and lights your way, don't expect that He will light up your *whole* journey—He might reveal just the next few steps. And don't imagine that His provision will arrive way ahead of time so you can stockpile it all until you're ready to use it. If you know the Old Testament story of the Israelites wandering in the desert for forty years, you'll remember God sent just enough manna—a grainlike food—for each day. (See Exodus 16.) If the Israelites tried to gather extra to save for the next day, the leftovers turned moldy—except for the day before the Sabbath, when they were permitted to collect a double portion that still would be fresh the next day. It's been my experience that God continues to provide just what His people need in the nick of time—not way ahead, as we organized, in-control people would like!

My favorite illustration of God's perfect timing is a story shared by Corrie ten Boom, the Dutch Christian concentration camp survivor whose family helped hide Jews from the Nazis during World War II. The conversation she relates took place when she was a little girl and her father tried to console her fears that she would be unprepared when she had to die someday:

> Father sat down on the edge of the narrow bed. "Corrie," he began gently, "when you and I go to Amsterdam—when do I give you your ticket?"
> I sniffed a few times, considering this.

"Why, just before we get on the train."

"Exactly. And our wise Father in heaven knows exactly when we're going to need things, too. Don't run out ahead of Him, Corrie. When the time comes that some of us will have to die, you will look into your heart and find the strength you need—just in time."[6]

"Don't run out ahead of Him."

What marvelous advice. God needs to go *before* us into each day. We don't yet have what we need to face all of our tomorrows, because we are not yet there. But every day as we come to our heavenly Father in prayer, He promises to guide us and provide for us in that minute, that hour, that day. I pray you'll have faith in Him, and I hope that this verse from Psalm 143:8 will be your prayer as you prepare to face another day without your loved one:

> Lord,
> Let me hear of your unfailing love each morning,
>   for I am trusting you.
> Show me where to walk,
>   for I give myself to you. Amen.

TAKE COMFORT: You don't have to fear tomorrow. . . . God is already there.

---

6. Corrie ten Boom, *The Hiding Place* (Grand Rapids: Chosen Books, 1971), 29.

13

Continuing On When It Doesn't Seem Possible

So when did you first hit the brick wall? You know, the place where it hurts so much you're certain continuing on without your loved one doesn't seem possible. Perhaps you hit it right away—especially if your loved one's death was completely unexpected or particularly violent or if your grief involves multiple losses. You may have crashed into it later when everyone else's life went back to "normal" and you realized that yours never would.

Regardless of your personal circumstances, you're at the wall when you feel that even if God is going on before you into each day, you simply don't have the strength to follow.

If you haven't hit it yet, chances are you're going to sometime—perhaps after the initial numbness wears off. And don't be surprised if you hit the wall *again*—even after you thought you were past it. Grief experts call it "the second wounding," and it occurs as the reality of your loss begins to sink in at an even deeper level.

But how do you continue on when it doesn't seem possible? Pull yourself up by your bootstraps? Get over it? Don't worry, be happy? Such shallow advice comes from those who haven't walked in your shoes.

I'd like to share three stories with you from grievers I know who *have* walked in shoes like yours. They have pressed on even though they all went through times when they thought they could not face another day of living. I hold them up, not as "model" grievers, but as fellow strugglers on their own unwanted journeys who, I believe, will give you hope that with God all things truly are possible.

My dear friend Joyce smacked up against her brick wall shortly after her son Tim, the next-to-youngest son of her six children, committed suicide just a month shy of his thirtieth birthday.

"When Tim took his life, I felt like he took mine, too," she recalls. "When the police called, I lost it. I screamed. I carried on. You just don't think you're going to hear something that terrible. I felt like I was dying— that I had lost a part of my body."

Joyce and her husband, Tod, say raising Tim always was a challenge. He was strong-willed even as a small child and never responded to the discipline techniques that had worked well on the other five children. As a handsome teenager, Tim was popular with the girls and a really good self-taught musician. But he had trouble concentrating at jobs and often made poor choices in his life. Depressed, divorced, and in debt, he made his last bad choice with a revolver in his hand on November 18, 2002.

It wasn't long before Joyce began to crack emotionally under the guilt she felt over numerous failed attempts to help Tim, and the grief she experienced over knowing he was gone forever from her life.

"I would sleep fourteen hours a day," she recalls. "Whenever I got a chance to nap, I did. I wanted nothing to do with reality. I didn't want to cook or bake or anything for my family. I even struggled to think what year it was."

Add to the equation the fact that Joyce was dealing with a second recurrence of breast cancer (first diagnosed in 1984) and the awful knowledge that her grandmother also had committed suicide many years before, and you can see why her brick wall was so hard and so high.

Continuing on with life just didn't seem possible.

But that was before Joyce and Tod got to see Luke 1:37 come true in their lives.

For nothing is impossible with God.

Slowly but steadily, with the right medication, good Christian counseling, and the healing touch of God, Joyce was able to push through her brick wall.

As I write, five years after Tim's death, Joyce still is fighting cancer, and both she and Tod still grieve the loss of their son. But Joyce is the person I probably look to most in my evening Cancer Prayer Support Group to encourage and pray for others who are in the storms of life. She has endless empathy for others who are in the pit of despair, and she willingly shares both the pain of— and the recovery from—her own depression.

"Grief makes you more dependent on God for all you face," Joyce says. "My relationship with God is so much stronger, and I trust in Him for everything—good or bad. I can even talk about Tim now and tell his story to other people who need to see how God can comfort."

Joyce is living proof that you will survive and that you can continue on with life. She has been to the brink and come back.

If anybody had a reason to give up on life and refuse to continue on, it was my friend Marge.[1] When I first heard the news about her family's horrible tragedy, I wondered how to even pray for her. You see, she had been critically injured in a drunk-driver crash,[2] which took the lives of her husband and their two grade-school daughters, as they were returning to Ohio from a family vacation in

1. My friend's name and a few minor details have been changed to protect her privacy.
2. Marge and many other victims of drunk drivers insist these incidents are crashes, *not* accidents, because the drunk drivers made a choice to get behind the wheel.

Florida. She was placed in a medically induced coma and on life support while doctors fought to save her. At that point, her church family contacted our church to solicit prayers on her behalf.

I wonder whether she would want me to pray that she lives or dies? I remember thinking at the time. I decided to pray that for her parents' sake she might live, and that if she did, God's miraculous grace would empower her to continue on even though it would seem impossible to do so.

Marge didn't hit the brick wall right away because her initial grief was gradual.

"As the narcotic dosages were decreased, I [began] to realize what had happened, what never would happen, and how drastically my reality had changed," she recalls. "I think I was blessed in some ways to be able to take doses of grief and go back into semiconsciousness."

When she finally fully emerged from the drugged fog, Marge says her grief was so intense that it was months before she could even concentrate on the simple task of reading a paragraph in a book.

"But I was blessed to have family, friends, and neighbors who provided physical and emotional support as needed with great sensitivity," she recounts. "This allowed me to find my own way at my own speed. No one pushed me to do anything I wasn't ready for."

Initially they managed some urgent decisions for her and postponed others until Marge was ready to participate in them. She believes the fact she was in a coma so long helped her family and friends process their own shock and grief somewhat before they began to come alongside her in her grief journey.

Ever so slowly she began to continue on with life.

"Thank goodness for the IRS," she says. "You won't hear many people say that, but it was the effort of preparing our annual tax return seven months after the crash that let me focus on a continuing thought process without emotion."

Marge pressed through her brick wall by reading a lot about grief as she tried to understand her own feelings and how she could begin to live again.

Now, almost twenty years since that terrible crash, which also killed the drunk driver and the driver's sister, Marge is repeatedly sought after to offer comfort to other grievers in similar situations. She volunteers with MADD, Mothers Against Drunk Driving, and is on its state board in Ohio.[3]

Because she has faced the unimaginable, she has a special sensitivity to deep grief and knows there are no words to make everything all right.

"I offer what I am able to others in grief, but I always feel disappointed that there is little I can offer but a willingness to listen," she says. "I believe that those who have experienced loss can *maybe* comprehend another's grief, but everyone grieves in different ways in their own time."

---

3. MADD is a nationwide organization of people determined to stop drunk driving and support the victims of drunk-driver crashes. See http://www.madd.org.

Marge professes "no profound insights" for fellow mourners, but she says she has learned that "God doesn't cause our grief or spare our grief but is with us to help bear us through it."

And I appreciate her candor when she acknowledges that, even though she has continued on with life, she still wishes it were different.

"Grief has given me a perspective on life's priorities, an appreciation of the significance of the moment, a delight in the distraction of the trivial, and a fearless-ness of death," she says. "But I would gladly give up all these insights to be fat, dumb, and happy and have my family back."

Marge's life is, I believe, a testimony to the God-given strength of the human spirit, which has enabled her to persevere through such an unthinkable loss and to give so many others hope that they can do the same.

While filling out tax forms helped Marge to press on with life, walking to the mailbox helped my friend Connie, whose husband, Brad, died while in Guatemala, to continue on with life after his sudden death.

"Every day I made myself do one thing to push through the pain," Connie recalls.

At first it was a daily walk to the mailbox.

"Brad always got the mail, and it was one more reminder of how much I hurt without him," she says.

Next she pushed through the pain of her brick wall by writing checks to pay some bills—another task Brad always did.

"I was emotionally exhausted after writing three checks," she remembers now with amazement at how low she was.

"I felt like I was someone on stage in a play I didn't want to be in. I didn't know my part and I wanted to get off the stage, but I couldn't," Connie explains.

Facing the Christmas season just three months after Brad's death was another brick wall for Connie.

"I felt terrible because I did not want to celebrate Jesus' birth because of Brad's death," she says.

A good friend gave her some insight that really helped ease her pain.

"He said, 'Do you want to know what Jesus is doing this Christmas season?'" Connie recalls. "'He's weeping. He's weeping with you.'"

That mental picture of Jesus weeping with her in her grief helped Connie believe her Lord truly did understand what she was feeling, even if no one else really could. She stopped worrying about all the holiday celebrations and instead prayed: *Just for today, I need to see Jesus. Just for today, I need to seek Jesus. Just for today, I need to serve Jesus.*

Connie's final push through the brick wall was the surrendering of her mind, which still had no answers to the whys of Brad's death.

"I realized that there are things I will never understand

and I don't have to understand and that I just need to let
go," Connie says.

> God, give us grace to accept with serenity the
> things that cannot be changed, courage to change
> the things that should be changed, and the wisdom
> to distinguish the one from the other.[4]

None of the grievers in this chapter could sit down
with you and tell you they understand why their loved
one had to die the way they did. They all still have
questions, hurts, and longings. And yet they all have
survived grief, though at times that didn't feel possible.

Their stories illustrate that you and I don't have to be
able to understand it all before we can continue on with
life. We can surrender the need to understand and accept
that we don't have the whole picture.

> *Now we see things imperfectly, like puzzling reflections
> in a mirror, but then we will see everything with perfect
> clarity. All that I know now is partial and incomplete,
> but then I will know everything completely just as God
> now knows me completely.* 1 CORINTHIANS 13:12

> *So we fix our eyes not on what is seen, but on what
> is unseen. For what is seen is temporary, but what is
> unseen is eternal.* 2 CORINTHIANS 4:18, NIV

---

4. Original poem attributed to Protestant theologian Reinhold Niebuhr
(1892–1971) and later adopted and slightly revised by Alcoholics
Anonymous as "The Serenity Prayer."

I love how Pastor Jon Walker explains this truth in one of his 2007 Purpose Driven Life daily e-mail devotionals.

"Read this sentence three times: 'The Truth is not dependent on my ability to understand what is going on.' (Okay, go back and really repeat it three times!) Let God interpret the facts; let him explain the situation. Meanwhile, focus on God and not on your *limited* ability to understand events or circumstances."[5]

Our views of life from inside a grief-storm are limited and distorted. We often cannot see or understand how what is happening could ever possibly be used as part of God's good plan for our lives. We don't have the big picture.

But accepting that we don't have the whole picture is not very comforting unless we also realize that God *does* have the whole picture *and* that He loves us greatly.

A few years ago on Mother's Day, our youngest daughter, Lindsey, who had just graduated from college (and as the daughter most like me, butted heads with me more than a few times during her teenage years), wrote me a note of appreciation that said in part: "I didn't always agree or understand when you said no to me, but I never doubted that you loved me."

That's what it means to trust. We choose never to doubt that God loves us even if we don't always agree or

---

5. "We Trust the Seasons, Why Not God?" October 30, 2007, http://www.purposedrivenlife.com.

understand when He says no to us. I often call to mind the words of Charles Haddon Spurgeon, the nineteenth-century British preacher, that have been popularized in a song by Babbie Mason: "God is too wise to be mistaken. God is too good to be unkind. So when you don't understand, when you can't see His plan, when you can't trace His hand—trust His heart."[6]

> *If God is for us, who can ever be against us? Since he did not spare even his own Son but gave him up for us all, won't he also give us everything else?* ROMANS 8:31-32

However, just knowing these two truths—that we don't have the whole picture but a God who loves us does—is not enough. We have to continue to walk by faith and not by sight—just as Joyce, Tod, Marge, Connie, and the other grievers I've written about are doing.

I'll be the first to admit that is not an easy task. Even if we're not from Missouri, we humans tend to be "show me" people. We want to see *first* and then believe. I am an extremely skeptical person (which makes me a great newspaper reporter but an annoying wife), and I *always* want the facts, the explanation, and the logic *before* I'll agree with just about anything.

But the Word of God, my compass in life and especially in storms, tells me that as believers we are different than others in this world because "we live by faith, not

---

6. Babbie Mason, "Trust His Heart" on *Timeless*, Spring Hill, 2001.

by sight."[7] Or as another translation puts it, "We live by believing and not by seeing."[8]

I must constantly remind myself that I don't need to see it all because God sees it all from the beginning of history to the end of time. As one writer explains: "Because we see only this sliver of time, we tend to view all of time through the same cracked and ill-fitting glasses. We forget that God is not bound by time. He exists outside of its minutes and millennia."[9]

He and only He has the big picture. We move ahead, not knowing for sure how it all will work out, but believing He does and will guide our way. I don't know how to say it any other way than we simply *walk by faith*.

> *Faith is the confidence that what we hope for will actually happen; it gives us assurance about things we cannot see.* HEBREWS 11:1

If you continue reading that chapter in Hebrews, you'll see great heroes of the faith—men and women (including grievers)—who believed that God was in control despite life's atrocities and trusted that His future heavenly blessings would more than make up for life's deep sorrows. Although they had great faith, they all died without seeing Jesus, the promised Messiah, who would take away their sins.

---

7. 2 Corinthians 5:7, NIV
8. 2 Corinthians 5:7, NLT
9. Taken from devotional published by the Outreach of Hope "God Keeps His Promises," 2001, http://www.outreachofhope.org/index.cfm/PageID/216/id/1691/cfid/2718392/cftoken/32326491/index.html.

All these people died still believing what God had promised them. They did not receive what was promised, but they saw it all from a distance and welcomed it. They agreed that they were foreigners and nomads here on earth. . . . But they were looking for a better place, a heavenly homeland. HEBREWS 11:13, 16

These heroes of the faith were disappointed by life, but they did not lose their faith because they believed this is *not* our real home—we were created for Heaven, not earth—even though we must spend a few years passing through here. Every deep disappointment here is designed to create a deeper longing in us for Heaven.

My heart weeps with yours because you have been forced to travel a journey you never would have chosen for yourself. The grief that follows having to say good-bye to loved ones—or even having to bury loved ones *without* a chance to say good-bye—feels unbearable.

"I've come to the conclusion it doesn't matter if you knew they were going to die and watched them suffer or you just lost them suddenly; it stinks and nothing prepares you for either," says my friend Gigi, whose parents drowned in the freak car accident.

It hurts to hit a brick wall, but it is *not* an impenetrable wall. It *is* possible for you to continue on the road where God is leading you. The next chapter in Hebrews tells us how:

> *And let us run with endurance the race God has set before us. We do this by keeping our eyes on Jesus, the champion who initiates and perfects our faith.*
> HEBREWS 12:1-2

With our eyes on Jesus, we can continue to walk by faith and not by sight. God's Word promises that He is able even if we are not. We don't have to pull ourselves up; His strength will hold us up. We don't have to get over our grief; His power will get us through it. We don't have to put on a happy face; His peace will fill us up.

> *The LORD gives strength to his people; the LORD blesses his people with peace.* PSALM 29:11, NIV

> *For all of God's promises have been fulfilled in Christ with a resounding "Yes!"* 2 CORINTHIANS 1:20

TAKE COMFORT: Remember the **ABC**s of grieving—**A**ccept you don't have the whole picture. **B**elieve God does and loves you greatly. **C**ontinue on by faith and not by sight.

14

KNOWING WHEN TO RELAX

The more I talk with my cousin Jim about his days of flying with an Air Force weather reconnaissance team, the more I believe that grieving is *a lot* like flying into a hurricane—both require an inordinate amount of trust.

Jim agrees with my observation and says it was difficult at first for him to trust he was going to be okay as his plane flew right into the eye of a storm.

"There's a lot of trust going on when you're going into harm's way," he explains. "You have to trust in the plane and the people who made it. You have to trust in the people who maintain the plane and that it won't fall apart. And you have to trust that the other crew members know what they're doing. And they all have to trust in you—that you will do the right thing too.

"But the more you do it, the more you know it's going to be okay," adds Jim, who has flown forty-four times into the eye of hurricanes and typhoons.

Jim says the scariest part of the team's mission to

gather weather data is the five or ten minutes just before the plane actually flies into the eye of the storm.

"You usually have to fly right through thunderstorms—which of course you normally would never do—and the turbulence is sometimes so severe you're really glad you're strapped into your seat," he explains.

But what happens next is so incredible it helps keep people like my cousin flying again and again into the eye of the storm.

"When you break through the eye wall, dramatically and suddenly the turbulence stops," Jim explains. "What was black and bleak is now sunny, quiet, beautiful, and really awe inspiring. There's blue sky above you, and you're like a little fish in the bottom of a bowl. You've found the exact calm center."

Now I fully realize that, unlike my cousin Jim, you have not *chosen* to fly into a hurricane. I also realize I can't change the fact that your life has been touched by an imperfect storm, that your world has fallen apart, and that you are trying to comprehend the incomprehensible. But I believe with all my heart that when God meets you in your grief, the Creator of the Universe is able to lead you to the exact calm center. I don't really understand how He does it any more than I understand how the middle of a hurricane can be beautifully quiet.

But Jim has been there so I believe him. The grievers in this book have been there, and I believe them, too.

Be still, and know that I am God! PSALM 46:10

That's where we find the exact calm center. It's the place where we can relax in the tight grip of a sovereign God. We relax *not* because everything is okay, but because we know the One who is in control . . . and will one day in Heaven make everything okay.

Here's how some other Bible versions translate Psalm 46:10:

> *Cease striving and know that I am God.*[1]

> *Desist, and know that I [am] God.*[2]

> *Let be and be still, and know (recognize and understand) that I am God.*[3]

> *Our God says, "Calm down, and learn that I am God!"*[4]

I've included all these translations because I'm such a word person and know that words can speak differently to each person. I'm praying that one of these translations has just the wording you need to hear.

Personally, I really like the very literal translation

1. New American Standard Bible
2. Young's Literal Translation
3. Amplified Bible
4. Contemporary English Version

to "cease striving." I tend to be an organized, driven person who tries really hard to get things worked out and doesn't do as well being still and "just" relaxing in God's control.

You may be like me or you may be someone who is *too* still and needs a heavenly kick to get you moving! Always being busy is not a healthy way to work through grief, but neither is always being alone and isolated. I believe we all need to find the right balance between at times pushing on (as those in the last chapter did) and at other times relaxing in His strength. It's tricky to always know which we need, but if each day we are reading our compass, God's Word, I believe the directions will be clear. For me, it is obvious that most of the time I need to cease striving and be still!

I have an incredible story to show how God recently drove home this point for me. Please hang in there with me as I share all the details because I believe the ending will amaze you, as it did me.

The story begins in March 2007 when I was teaching Bill Hybels's book *Just Walk Across the Room* in one of our adult classes at church. Hybels suggested we contact and thank the person who "walked across the room" and first invited us to faith. I knew I needed to contact Dave Sheldon, a guy at *the* Ohio State University (we were taught to say it that way!) who invited my roommate Jackie and me to a Campus Crusade for Christ meeting in January 1972. When he invited us, I wasn't at all interested in the meeting or in spiritual matters but said I'd go because I didn't want my roommate to look "holier" than me (yes, I am a competitive person!).

That night I surrendered leadership of my life to Jesus and have never looked back. Although Dave and I were friends for a while before I moved away, I'd never really thanked him for taking the small—but crucial—step of inviting me to a deeper faith. Now, I thought he probably would be excited to hear all God had done in my life in the three decades since he had walked across my apartment room.

So I came home that Sunday and prayed God would help me find Dave Sheldon. I then began searching for him on the Internet. The last I knew, he had been a pastor living in Columbus, Ohio. I searched the OSU alumni directory and online Columbus phone books but found no Dave Sheldons. I broadened my search to all of Ohio and even called a couple of numbers, but I still couldn't find him. I searched church Web sites, but to no avail. As an ex-reporter, I pride myself in being able to locate hard-to-find people, but after a couple of hours, I finally gave up.

Okay, God, I thought you would want me to find Dave Sheldon. I asked You to help me find him. All I wanted to do was thank him and tell him all You've done for me. But if You want me to wait until Heaven to thank him, then I guess that's what I'll have to do.

End of praying, end of trying. I didn't think about Psalm 46:10 right then, but I basically ceased striving and acknowledged that God was God and He didn't have to help me find Dave Sheldon.

Fast-forward nine months to Christmastime when my husband, our eldest daughter, Danielle, and I visited my parents in Ashland, Ohio (about one hour north of Columbus). While we were there, we wanted to see a particular movie, so we told Danielle to pick a day, a theater, and a time for us to go. She researched our options online and chose an old theater right in town, only to later discover that the movie would be shown upstairs and there was no elevator for my mom. So Danielle chose a new time and a new theater in Mansfield, about thirty minutes away. We went out to lunch before the movie. Afterward, I wanted to go back to our motel to get my buttered-popcorn jelly beans, but Ralph said he didn't think we'd have time. (Yes, I know it's "illegal" to sneak them into a theater, but the candy has so many fewer calories than real buttered popcorn.)

Amazingly, I didn't argue with Ralph about going back for them (a small miracle in itself). Instead we drove to Mansfield and found the new theater—arriving about forty minutes early! Thankfully, I didn't whine that we would have had time to get the jelly beans (another miracle). We bought our show tickets and discussed how to kill some time before the movie. My husband's new GPS told us there was a Wal-Mart nearby, so we decided to go there and pick up some things my mom needed. But after the GPS calculated our arrival time, I decided we probably didn't have enough time. I looked around and noticed a new Bed Bath & Beyond store and suggested we take my mom there so she could see the dishes in our youngest daughter's wedding registry.

With my mom on my arm, we walked very slowly up the store aisle and looked at Lindsey's registry items. After about twenty-five minutes, I realized we needed to get back to the theater. I started to take my mom back down the same aisle because it was the fastest way out, but a little voice in my head said, *Why don't you relax and take her down another aisle so she can enjoy looking at some different things on the way out?* So we walked to the far side of the store and down the last aisle. Near the end of it, we stopped at a big display of Ohio State paraphernalia. (Stores in Pennsylvania, where I now live, never have such *wonderful* displays of my alma mater!)

A man I didn't recognize was standing near the display. He said to me: "Lynn?"

I answered yes. He looked quizzically at my face and said, "You *are* Lynn, aren't you?"

Again I said yes while thinking: *I've finally been recognized by a complete stranger who read one of my books—this is so cool!* (Afterward my mother and Danielle both confessed they thought the same thing!)

Then the man said with a big smile: "Dave Sheldon."

I was speechless as I hugged him for dear life. Finally, I managed to tell him that I had prayed to find him because I wanted to thank him for inviting me to the meeting that changed my life. We talked for a few moments before exchanging e-mail addresses. I learned he is no longer a pastor in Columbus but lives in Mansfield and was in Bed, Bath & Beyond killing time with his son-in-law while his wife and daughters were at a nearby Target store. I marvel that Dave last saw me thirty-four years ago when I was twenty years old yet still recognized me. (I knew not changing my hairstyle would pay off someday!)

Be still, and know that I am God!

If I initially had found Dave Sheldon on the Internet that day I prayed to find him, I would have been very happy. But God had a much better plan. He somehow, someway managed to put Dave Sheldon and me in the same state, the same city, the same store, the same aisle, at the same display, at the exact same moment in time. When I put my head on my pillow that night, I couldn't stop smiling. As I said my prayers, I was very still and I knew without a shadow of a doubt that He was God.

The word translated *still* in Psalm 46:10 is the Hebrew word *harpu*. I'm no Hebrew scholar, but I did some research and found it conveys the idea of being weak, letting go, surrendering, or releasing. It's the opposite of striving with our arms up, ready to fight or at least defend ourselves. When we are *harpu*, our arms are at our sides, relaxed.

A great story in the Old Testament illustrates this idea. It's found in 2 Chronicles 20. The short background of the story is that the Jewish king Jehoshaphat was told that some great armies were coming to attack him. His response was not atypical from what ours might be—he "was terrified by this news and begged the LORD for guidance" (2 Chronicles 20:3). Shortly, God answered his prayer by sending His Spirit to speak through one of the king's men:

> He said, "Listen, all you people of Judah and Jerusalem! Listen, King Jehoshaphat! This is what the LORD says: Do not be afraid! Don't be discouraged by this mighty army, for the battle is not yours, but God's. Tomorrow, march out against them. You will find them coming up through the ascent of Ziz at the end of the valley that opens into the wilderness of Jeruel. But you will not even need to fight. Take your positions; then stand still and watch the LORD's victory. He is with you, O people of Judah and Jerusalem. Do not be afraid or discouraged. Go out against them tomorrow, for the LORD is with you!" 2 CHRONICLES 20:15-17

The king and his people believed God and began to worship Him, praise Him, and sing to Him. At the very moment they did this, the Bible says God caused the approaching armies to fight among themselves and kill each other. The Israelites won the battle without a fight because God fought for them.

Logically, standing still does not sound like a good way to win a battle. But then God's ways are not our ways, are they? The armies coming against Jehoshaphat were way too large and powerful for his army to defeat. The situation was hopeless from his perspective—but it was hope-filled from God's vantage point.

I know grieving is a hard battle. Perhaps at times you feel the grief is too large and powerful for you and your situation is hopeless. But it is not really your battle— it is the Lord's. Sometimes He will fight through you (when you need to push on through the pain) and other times He will fight for you. At those times, you can do as Jehoshaphat and the Israelites did: stand still and watch the Lord's victory. We can relax as Psalm 46:10 suggests because God is at work on our behalf. And when our prayers aren't answered as quickly as we had wished— like my prayer to find Dave Sheldon—we still can relax, knowing that God is in control.

What a relief to know the Lord goes before us into each new day, so we do not need to be afraid or discouraged. We can cease from striving and believe that, just like God knew how to lead me to Dave Sheldon, He knows how to go before you and guide your steps.

The Bible doesn't say: "God helps those who help themselves." Its message is the opposite: God helps the helpless.

The LORD lifts up those who are weighed down.
PSALM 146:8

You hear, O LORD, the desire of the afflicted; you encourage them, and you listen to their cry.
PSALM 10:17, NIV

For the LORD comforts his people and will have compassion on his afflicted ones. ISAIAH 49:13, NIV

"So as your world crumbles around you, the call from Scripture is: don't flinch in faith in God. Stand still—not because of a self-made confidence, not because you are the most composed person in the face of disaster, not because 'you've seen it all.' Be still because of what you know about God."[5]

Joe Stowell, former president of Moody Bible Institute, explains that Psalm 46:10 "is not saying that we cease from striving because we know how it is going to work out, but we know the God who will work it out. Knowing God is better than knowing outcomes."[6]

There's a beautiful song by Reuben Morgan called "Still," and the chorus keeps running through my mind:

When the oceans rise and thunders roar,
I will soar with You above the storm.
Father, You are king over the flood.
I will be still and know You are God.[7]

5. Jason Jackson, "Be Still and Know That I Am God," *Christian Courier*, February 27, 2006.
6. "Trusting God in Times of Crisis," available at http://www.preachingtodaysermons.com/stowjostrusg.html.
7. "Still," words and music by Reuben Morgan © 2002 Reuben Morgan and Hillsong Publishing (admin. in the U.S. and Canada by Integrity's Hosanna! Music)/ASCAP c/o Integrity Media, Inc., 1000 Cody Road, Mobile, AL 36695. All rights reserved. International copyright secured. Used by permission.

My prayer for you is that you know God well enough to really trust Him. I don't mean know *about* Him intellectually, but know Him *personally* as your heavenly Father who loves you with an everlasting love. If you're ever unsure about the depth of that love, remember: you didn't have a choice about your loved one's death, but He did have a choice about His Son's.

> *For God loved the world so much that he gave his one and only Son, so that everyone who believes in him will not perish but have eternal life.* JOHN 3:16

What great *grief* the Father must have felt as He watched His only Son tortured on that wooden cross. What lavish love to *willingly* allow His Son to die. What supreme sorrow He must feel when we take His sacrifice lightly.

If you truly appreciate that sacrifice He made for you, I urge you to get to know your heavenly Father in a deeper way. Feed your spirit with His Word. Pour out your heart at His feet. Praise Him with others who share your faith. Live a holy life that pleases Him. Make knowing Him and making Him known to others the goal of your life.

Chances are I don't know you and we never will meet. But whether I know you or not, I certainly don't know exactly how God is going to work out your grief-storm for you. And I definitely don't know the outcomes of your life.

But I do know God.

I know His Word is as trustworthy as the magnetic
poles of the earth.
I know He feels your pain when your world falls
apart.
I know He can find a friend who understands your
sorrow.
I know He won't let your loved one's memory die.
I know He will hold you up so you can let down
and let go.
I know His strength will carry you even when you
face the incomprehensible.
I know He will enable you to survive this imperfect
storm.
I know His "windows" can take any angry rocks
you throw.
I know He wants to use you to comfort others.
I know He can create beauty from ashes, turn
mourning into dancing, and change weeping
into joy.
I know His promise of Heaven changes everything
for believers.
I know you don't have to fear tomorrow because
God already is there.
I know He will empower you to continue on when
it doesn't seem possible.
I know He wants to lead you to the exact calm cen-
ter where you relax in His divine control.

So go ahead and let Him be the unfalteringly faithful God, willing to strengthen you for any and every circumstance. Go ahead and let Him be the supremely sovereign God, wise enough to know how and when to answer any and every prayer. Go ahead and let Him be the absolutely awesome God that He is, powerful enough to comfort you at any and every level.

Be still and let God meet you in your grief.

TAKE COMFORT: Knowing God is better than knowing anything else.

Grief Books for Adults

In addition to this book, *When God & Grief Meet* (Tyndale, 2009),
I recommend the following resources:

Confessions of a Grieving Christian by Zig Ziglar (Broadman & Holman,
2004). Lessons learned by this well-known motivational speaker after
the loss of his adult daughter.

A Decembered Grief by Harold Ivan Smith (Beacon Hill Press of Kansas City,
1999). Living with loss while others are celebrating.

Don't Sing Songs to a Heavy Heart by Kenneth C. Haugk (Stephen
Ministries, 2004). How to relate to those who are suffering.

Everyday Comfort: Meditations for Seasons of Grief by Randy Becton (Baker
Books, 2006). Thirty daily devotions to help navigate through heartache.

Experiencing Grief by H. Norman Wright (B&H Publishing Group, 2004).
A short book helping readers deal with the five stages of grief.

Finding Your Way after the Suicide of Someone You Love by David B. Biebel and
Suzanne L. Foster (Zondervan, 2005). A compassionate and practical guide
that addresses the intensely personal issues of suicide for those left behind.

Forgiving God by Carla Killough McClafferty (Discovery House Publishers,
2000). Written by a mother who lost her young son and attempts to forgive
a loving God who did not answer her prayers for her son.

Getting to the Other Side of Grief: Overcoming the Loss of a Spouse by
Susan J. Zonnebelt-Smeenge and Robert C. De Vries (Baker Books, 1998).
Written by two widowed persons on "overcoming" the loss of a spouse.

A Gift of Mourning Glories: Restoring Your Life After Loss by Georgia Shaffer
(Vine Books, 2000). An excellent book on restoring your life after all kinds
of loss.

God on the Witness Stand: Questions Christians Ask in Personal Tragedy by
Daniel T. Hans (Baker Publishing Group, 1989). A pastor whose little girl
died from a brain tumor answers the questions Christians ask during personal tragedy. (Hans also authored the booklet *When a Child Dies* [Desert
Ministries, 1998]).

Good Grief by Granger E. Westberg (Augsburg Fortress, 2005). Since its first
edition in 1962, this booklet has become a standard resource for people grieving losses. Written by a pioneer in the holistic health movement.

A Grace Disguised: How the Soul Grows through Loss by Jerry Sittser (Zondervan, 2005). This book, written by a man who lost his wife, daughter, and mother in one car accident, plumbs the depths of sorrows. His hope-filled conclusion is that it's not what happens to us that matters so much as what happens in us.

Grief (Discovery House Publishers, 2006). Sixty daily devotions on the topic of grief taken from *Our Daily Bread* magazine.

A Grief Observed by C. S. Lewis (HarperOne, 2001). Lewis wrote this near the end of his life after a dramatic and unexpected romance ended in the death of his new wife from cancer. Very personal, raw emotions emerge as he struggles with grief and his Christian faith.

The Grief Recovery Handbook: The Action Program for Moving Beyond Death, Divorce, and Other Losses by John W. James and Russell Friedman (HarperCollins, 1998). A wonderful resource in dealing with unresolved grief.

A Grief Sanctified: Through Sorrow to Eternal Hope by J. I. Packer and Richard Baxter (Crossway Books, 2002). A memoir by Baxter about the loss of his wife, with beautiful insights added by Packer.

Grieving: Our Path Back to Peace by James R. White (Bethany House, 1997). An insightful Bible teacher, counselor, and chaplain shares how to find hope in the midst of hurt.

Grieving the Loss of a Loved One by Kathe Wunnenberg (Zondervan, 2000). A devotional companion (with space for writing your own thoughts) by a woman who experienced three miscarriages and the death of her infant son.

He Cares New Testament with Psalms and Proverbs (Tyndale, 2007). Inspirational commentary by Lynn Eib. Filled with encouragement, guidance, and answers for heavy hearts or questioning minds. Suitable for those dealing with chronic and/or serious illness, as well as grievers. Offered in the easy-to-understand New Living Translation, with special helps for those not familiar with reading the Bible.

Heaven by Randy Alcorn (Tyndale, 2004). The best book on Heaven I've ever read. Written by the founder and director of Eternal Perspectives Ministries. Readers will come away with an understanding of and a longing for Heaven like never before.

Holding On to Hope by Nancy Guthrie (Tyndale, 2002). A pathway through suffering to the heart of God, written by a woman whose infant daughter and son died from a rare genetic condition.

Jonathan, You Left Too Soon by David B. Biebel (Baker Publishing Group, 1997). Intensely personal story of how one man, as a father and a pastor, came to terms with the sudden death of his three-year-old son.

Let Me Grieve but Not Forever: A Journey Out of the Darkness of Loss by Verdell Davis (Thomas Nelson, 1994). A memoir from the personal journals of the author after the death of her husband.

Letters to Darcy by Tracy Ramos (Tyndale House, 2009). A mother's heartfelt letters to her unborn child with a rare genetic syndrome who lived only two weeks after birth. The author recommends www.HeavenlyAngelsInNeed.com and www.NowILayMeDownToSleep.com for those who have lost a baby before or shortly after birth.

Making Sense Out of Suffering by Peter Kreeft (Servant Books, 1986). A philosophy professor at Boston College wrestles with God as he tries to make sense of the pain and suffering in his own life, as well as in the world.

Mourning into Dancing by Walter Wangerin Jr. (Zondervan, 1992). An in-depth look at grief and loss and the hope of restored relationships.

Reflections of a Grieving Spouse by H. Norman Wright (Harvest House, 2009). A noted grief and trauma counselor who lost his wife to cancer shares a compassionate and practical guide for surviving the loss of the one you love.

Restore My Soul: A Grief Companion by Lorraine Peterson (NavPress, 2000). A short chapter for each day of the month offering ways to cope with life. Each also includes Scripture readings and a suggested prayer.

A Sacred Sorrow: Reaching Out to God in the Lost Language of Lament by Michael Card (NavPress, 2005). Author, musician, and Bible teacher Michael Card takes the reader through the Scriptures as a way to better understand God's desire for us to pour out our hearts to Him, whether in joy or pain.

Safe in the Arms of God: Truth from Heaven about the Death of a Child by John MacArthur (Thomas Nelson, 2003). This renowned Bible teacher tackles the question of infant death (in the womb or after birth), using many Scriptures to bring truth and consolation.

A Severe Mercy by Sheldon Vanauken (HarperOne, 1987). While studying at Oxford, the author and his wife, Davy, became friends with C. S. Lewis, who helped them come to faith. A beautiful love story of faith, intellect, ideology, and lessons learned from suffering after Davy's sudden death.

The Shack by William P. Young (Windblown Media, 2007). A provocative novel that wrestles with this timeless question: "Where is God in the midst of unspeakable pain?" A hope-filled book for any griever but especially comforting to those who have lost a young child or loved one to an act of violence.

Tear Soup by Pat Schwiebert and Chuck DeKlyen (Grief Watch, 1999). This wonderful picture book affirms the bereaved, educates the nonbereaved, and is a building block for children understanding grief. Excellent for adults and children. Also available on CD and video at www.griefwatch .com/tearsoup.

Tracks of a Fellow Struggler: Living and Growing through Grief by John R. Claypool (Morehouse Publishing, 2004). Adapted from four sermons this pastor-author gave about his family's journey through suffering and grief after his daughter's diagnosis and subsequent death from leukemia. A classic that has sold more than one million copies.

The View from a Hearse by Joseph Bayly (David C. Cook Publishing, 1973). This book is out of print, but you can still find used copies online. The author lost three sons at three different times and knows firsthand the devastation of parental grief.

When a Loved One Dies by Philip W. Williams (Augsburg Fortress, 1995). A short book of daily meditations for the journey through grief.

When God & Cancer Meet by Lynn Eib (Tyndale, 2002). True stories of hope and healing, which will bless not only those who are facing cancer, but those who have lost a loved one to the disease.

When God Doesn't Answer Your Prayer by Jerry Sittser (Zondervan, 2003). Explores the mysteries and paradoxes of unanswered prayer.

When God Weeps by Joni Eareckson Tada and Steven Estes (Zondervan, 1997). An excellent scriptural look at God's intentions for us in our pain and suffering.

When Life Is Changed Forever by the Death of Someone Near by Rick Taylor (Harvest House, 1993). An honest journey into the depths of God's love for all those who have experienced the complicated and often conflicting emotions brought on by a loved one's death. Written by a pastor who lost a young son in a drowning accident.

When Your Family's Lost a Loved One by David and Nancy Guthrie (Focus on the Family, 2008). Written by a couple who lost two infants to a rare genetic disorder, these honest reflections explore the family dynamics involved in grief and provide helpful insights into how a family can pull together rather than be pulled apart after the death of a loved one.

Why Me? A Doctor Looks at the Book of Job by Diane M. Komp (InterVarsity Press, 2001). This professor emeritus of pediatric oncology at Yale University School of Medicine addresses deep questions on suffering and grief with sensitivity and divine truth.

The Wounded Healer by Henri Nouwen (Doubleday, 1979). Fresh insights into how our own woundedness can help us offer strength and healing to others who are grieving.

GRIEF BOOKS FOR KIDS

Children and Grief by Joey O'Connor (Revell, 2004). Written from a Christian perspective to help children of all ages understand death.

Heaven for Kids by Randy Alcorn (Tyndale, 2006). Answers kids will understand based on the book *Heaven*. Written in an easy-to-use Q&A format, the book covers the eternal topics kids wonder about.

It's Okay to Cry: A Parent's Guide to Helping Children through the Losses of Life by H. Norman Wright (WaterBrook Press, 2004). Practical helps for parents explaining the symptoms of loss and unresolved grief so parents can walk with their children on this journey. Includes help for all losses, not just death.

Love Sick: Teens Reflect on Growing Up with a Parent Who Has Cancer (CancerConnected.com, 2008). Teens who have lost a parent to cancer will discover others who share their deep feelings.

Saying Goodbye When You Don't Want To by Martha Bolton (Vine Books, 2002). For teens dealing with the death of relatives or friends, as well as other non-death-related grief.

Someday Heaven by Larry Libby and Wayne McLoughlin (Zonderkidz, 2001). Provides biblically based answers on a topic that is not always easy to explain to a young child.

Someone I Loved Died (Please Help Me, God) by Christine Harder Tangvald (Chariot Victor Publishing, 1988). Includes a faith-parenting guide and helpful, personal activities.

Tear Soup by Pat Schwiebert and Chuck DeKlyen (Grief Watch, 1999). This wonderful picture book affirms the bereaved, educates the nonbereaved, and is a building block for children understanding grief. Excellent for adults and children. Also available in CD and video at www.griefwatch.com/tearsoup.

What Happens When We Die? by Carolyn Nystrom and Eira Reeves, Mini Book Edition (Moody Press, 1992) A simple yet profound book showing younger children some of the reasons people die and what God has in store for us in Heaven.

GRIEF CARE ORGANIZATIONS AND RESOURCES

Abbey Press. Grief support kits and inexpensive booklets that can be used for grief support group discussion. **www.carenotes.com**

American Foundation for Suicide Prevention. Programs for survivors of suicide loss; contact them at (888) 333-AFSP or **www.afsp.org**

The Compassionate Friends. National support group for bereaved parents, siblings, and grandparents who have experienced the death of a child at any age. 877-969-0010. **www.compassionatefriends.org**

The Dougy Center. National center for grieving children and families. Provides peer support groups for grieving children at no charge. **www.dougy.org**

griefHaven. Support and resources for families who have lost a child. **www.griefhaven.org**

GriefNet. An Internet community offering dozens of e-mail support groups at **www.griefnet.org**. Their sister site, **http://kidsaid.com**, is a safe place for children to share and help each other deal with grief.

Grief Recovery. Workbooks, personal workshops, and other resources to aid in the grieving process. **www.grief-recovery.com**

GriefShare. Seminars and support groups from a Christian perspective meeting throughout the United States, Canada, and in more than ten other countries. Daily devotions and resources available at **www.griefshare.org**.

Grief Watch. Resources for bereaved families and professional caregivers, including those who have lost an infant before or after birth. 503-284-7426. **www.griefwatch.com**

Living with Loss. A quarterly magazine of hope and healing for body, mind, and spirit. **www.livingwithloss.com**

Endurance with Jan and Dave Dravecky. Resources from a Christian perspective offering guidance and support for those who suffer, including those who have lost a loved one to cancer. Prayer support, online devotionals, and professional resources. 719-481-3528. **www.endurance.org**

Stephen Ministries. A one-to-one caring ministry by trained lay ministers in local Christian congregations. Devotions, as well as grief resources and training opportunities for Stephen Ministers, are available online. **www.stephenministries.org**

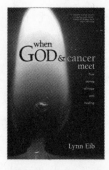
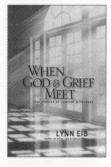
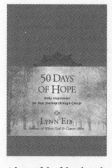
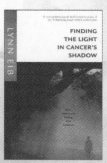
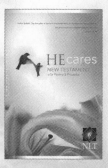